THE
WATERFALL
DIET

THE
WATERFALL
DIET

LOSE UP TO **14 POUNDS** IN 7 DAYS
BY CONTROLLING **FLUID RETENTION**

LINDA LAZARIDES

PIATKUS

Acknowledgements

I would like to thank the following people for their help with this book. First, my patients, who showed me what a widespread problem fluid retention is, and how little it is understood. Second, those doctors and scientists who have found evidence that it is a nutrition-related problem and have tried to tell the world by writing up their work for medical journals. And, finally, Dr Jean Monro for her ever-generous help and support, Health Interlink Ltd and Great Smokies Laboratory for educating me on liver function, Wainwright Churchill for e-mailing me details of the research into bias against natural medicine, Mr Y. Pang of Payden's chemist, Hailsham, for his assistance with the pharmaceutical section, Carolyn Gibbs for providing many excellent recipes, Dr Judith Casley-Smith and Dr Robert Woodward for information on coumarin, Pennie Hayes for looking after my office, Rita Quinlan of the Nutrition Centre, Heathfield for assistance with locating health food products, and Rachel Winning of Piatkus Books for her editorial help and advice.

© 1999 by Linda Lazarides

First published in 1999 by
Judy Piatkus (Publishers) Ltd
5 Windmill Street, London W1P 1HF

The moral right of the author has been asserted

A catalogue record for this book is available from the British Library

ISBN 0 7499 2025 4

Designed by Sara Kidd

Data capture by Action Publishing Technology, Gloucester
Printed and bound in Great Britain by
The Bath Press, Bath

Contents

How To Use this Book

Fluid retention has many causes. Chapter 1 aims to help you find out whether you might have this condition, and Chapters 2–8 provide questionnaires and information to help you find out *why* you have it. For some people the cause is relatively straightforward, like a food allergy or protein deficiency. Once you eliminate the food that is causing the allergy, you can lose a lot of weight very quickly – up to 14 pounds in the first week. For other people the cause may be quite complex, involving several body systems, so do fill in the questionnaire at the beginning of each chapter in case more than one chapter applies to you.

Each of these chapters explains one of the body systems which can be involved, what can make it go wrong, and how fluid retention can result. One or more case studies help to illustrate the point. The panels of text at the end of chapters contain more in-depth information, and can be skipped if you prefer. Once you have read Chapters 1–8, list which causes of fluid retention apply to you; several may be involved. You will need this list when you begin Phase III of the Waterfall Diet.

Chapter 9, the diet itself, contains the information you need to put right what has caused your fluid retention. The diet itself is in three parts: Phases I and II are for everyone, regardless of your type of fluid retention, and Phase III is adjusted to your particular type(s). Following Phase I of the diet can also help to confirm whether or not you have fluid retention, if your answers to the questionnaire in Chapter 1 have left you feeling unsure. If you lose weight on Phase I but not on an ordinary calorie-controlled diet then you probably did have fluid retention, especially if you have a high score in one or more of the questionnaires in Chapters 2–8.

Once you progress to Phase III, on p. 166 you will find a table which tells you how to adjust the diet to your particular type(s) of fluid retention. If you were retaining fluid, you should by this time have lost most of it. Phase III of the diet is designed to prevent it from returning, while at the same time allowing you plenty of treats.

Note for Doctors and Dieticians

As medicine becomes more and more specialized it is inevitable that the 'big picture' represented by the enormously complex human body must become more and more elusive. But without seeing more of the big picture, it is difficult to give patients what they really want: to be well again. Instead, medicine is resorting to superficial palliatives: painkillers, anti-inflammatories, steroid creams and antidepressants, and the removal of body parts if they become too painful or dysfunctional. Chronic diseases, ailments and disabilities are now damaging the lives of about one third of the UK population.

Dietetics is little better, being taught as the scientific study of food and considered irrelevant to the vast majority of diseases. Television dieticians are recommending junk food to children who are already eating dangerously high quantities of it.

This book approaches a very common and distressing medical problem – idiopathic oedema – by using a synthesis of knowledge from many disciplines, including lymphology, immunology and endocrinology. It demonstrates that trying to see more of the big picture can open up a whole new world to the health practitioner – a world where symptoms and lifestyle become clues and the doctor becomes a detective tracking down causes of ill health. While explained in terms simple enough for the lay person to understand, this book is nevertheless full of medical information based on research published in peer-review journals.

Most of your patients will welcome this highly practical treatment protocol for obesity that does not respond to calorie-controlled diets or to the treatment of recognized metabolic disorders. If you send a stamped, addressed envelope to the address on p. 210, I will be glad to supply all NHS public clinics and health centres with a single, condensed information and diet sheet which can be photocopied for your patients' use. I would also welcome receiving the results of any clinical audits from the use of the Waterfall Diet in the treatment of obesity or idiopathic oedema. Both NHS and private clinics may apply to me for prices of low-cost pamphlets giving details of the diet and information about it, supplied in bulk.

Linda Lazarides

CHAPTER

Could Fluid Be Your Problem?

To be able to sit on the loo and urinate away up to 20 lbs of excess body weight in a few days probably sounds like something out of your wildest dreams. Yet many people have done it and been delighted with the results. Right now, scientists all over the world are looking at the causes of fluid retention and helping us to understand how it can affect our body weight. If you can answer yes to two or more of the following questions, it is very likely that you too may be able to urinate some of your body weight away.

Fluid Retention Questionnaire

- Have you worked hard to slim using conventional methods, and found that you cannot get below a certain weight even if you persevere for months or years?
- Press a fingernail firmly into your thumb-pad. Does it stay dented for more than a second or two?
- Press the tip of your finger into the inside of your shinbone. Can your finger make a dent?
- Do your ankles ever swell up?
- Does your shoe size seem to increase as you get older?
- Do your rings sometimes seem not to fit you any more?
- Is your tummy often tight and swollen?
- If you are a woman, do you often suffer from breast tenderness?
- Does your weight ever fluctuate by several pounds within the space of only twenty-four hours?

Why Fat Loss Diets May Fail

At present most so-called slimming experts have little to offer us other than 'fat loss' diets. These diets are based on the assumption that all our excess weight is body fat, and purely depends on how many calories we consume and how many we burn off as exercise. Yet the human body is far more complex than this. For instance;

- How fast or slow is your metabolism?
- What part do hormones play in controlling your weight?
- Do you eat like a sparrow, run for hours every week, yet still not lose weight?

You will still get the same answer from your dietician: 'Eat fewer calories and exercise more'.

The usual attitude that 'it just takes a little bit of effort' makes people with a weight problem very angry when they have worked hard at dieting and got nowhere. Dozens have consulted me on the verge of tears, torn between feeling desperately guilty that they just *couldn't* eat any less, and feeling extremely angry that their doctor or dietician would not believe how few calories they were eating. 'My doctor more or less accused me of stuffing myself with chocolate bars and just not admitting it', is a comment I have heard over and over again.

If you have this problem, you already know how frustrating it is to spend a fortune on regular gym sessions, to feel constantly depressed from eating a very low-calorie diet lacking in all your favourite foods, to get up early to go jogging before work – and then to be accused of lying because none of this is getting you down to your target weight. It is not unusual for some people actually to *gain* weight on the calorie-controlled diets which doctors or dieticians give them, because they had previously been following a diet of only 500–800 calories a day. Again, it is hard to make anyone believe this.

If this sounds like you, then it is *not* excess fat that is making you overweight.

What is body fat?

The reason why is fairly clear. Body fat is a form of stored energy. As you may know, energy is measured in calories: when we say that a certain amount of a food provides us with one calorie, we mean that this food can yield enough energy to raise the temperature of one gram of water by one degree Celsius. One kcal or Calorie (with a capital C) is equal to 1000 calories.

Calories which we have absorbed from our food, but which remain unused because our level of physical activity is too low, go into storage as body fat. So if we reduce our calorie intake enough for our normal level of physical activity to burn up all the calories that we eat, plus some of the calories that we have stored away as fat, we will start losing fat. If at the same time we increase our level of physical activity by exercising, stored fat will be lost even more quickly. So by all the laws of science, it stands to reason that, if a calorie-controlled diet is only partially effective, it is not your body fat that is making you overweight.

Hormone imbalance

Sometimes, of course, your hormones are to blame. For instance, a thyroid deficiency will cause your metabolism to slow down – your body fat accumulates more easily and burns off more slowly. But your doctor will normally be able to rule out a problem like this with a test and give you thyroid hormone supplements if necessary.

The role of water

One factor which is very rarely taken into account when you are given a weight loss programme is water. Did you know that your body actually consists of 50–60 per cent water?

Water is found both inside and outside our cells. It forms part of our blood, helping to carry our blood cells around the body and keeping important nutrients in solution so that they can be taken up by tissues such as glands, bone and muscle. Even our organs and muscles are mostly water.

Your body uses a complex system of hormones and hormone-like substances called prostaglandins to keep its volume of fluid at a constant level. So if one day you drink a lot more water or other fluid than usual, you will not end up weighing more; your kidneys will quickly be stimulated to excrete the excess as urine. Likewise, if you do not get enough to drink, your body will hold on to its precious fluids and you will urinate much less than usual.

But what if this system goes wrong, and fluid accumulates instead of being excreted? If you have no particular medical symptoms the chances are that mild fluid retention, amounting to, say, 7–20 lbs (3–9 kg) of body weight, would not be recognized as fluid. You or your doctor would simply believe that you are overweight due to eating too much or not exercising enough.

How and Where Does Fluid Accumulate?

If you have great difficulty in reaching a normal weight, and if your doctor cannot find any medical explanation, the chances are that your fluid balance mechanisms have gone wrong and you are not excreting enough water. Fluid retention means that, instead of consisting of 50–60 per cent water, your body weight may be 65 per cent water or even more. (The terms 'water retention' and 'fluid retention' are more or less synonymous. Pure water does not occur in the body – it is always mixed with other substances.)

Fluid retention is usually said to result from changes in the pressure inside the capillaries – the smallest blood vessels in the body – or changes in the permeability (leakiness) of the capillary walls. These changes cause fluid to leak into the surrounding tissues, where it can accumulate in the tissue spaces around and between your body's cells instead of being carried to your veins and finally syphoned off by your kidneys into your bladder, along with waste products.

The reason why fluid retention can be so hard to diagnose is that almost all your body's tissues have plenty of capacity to hold a little more water without looking abnormal. For example, excess fluid could be making your tummy look rather large. When you pinch it, you can feel its normal covering of fat. You may easily believe that your tummy's size is due to this fat. But if you lose your excess fluid your tummy may subside and flatten, so that you can see you have no more fat there than on the rest of your body. (Of course, a tummy with slack, poorly toned muscles due to lack of exercise can also look big. Good muscle tone is very important for maintaining a good figure.)

Medical books usually quote the following as causes of the capillary changes which can lead to fluid retention:

- Cirrhosis of the liver
- Heart or kidney failure
- Histamine release (often allergy-related)
- Obstruction of the lymphatic system
- Starvation
- Thrombosis

But many less daunting factors, such as salt retention, hormonal imbalances and vitamin or mineral deficiencies can encourage fluid retention, and these are discussed in Chapters 2–8. Fluid can also accumulate in cavities within the body, for instance in the abdominal cavity which holds your organs of digestion and absorption.

Could You Be Retaining Fluid?

How likely is it that our fluid balance could go wrong? And how will you know if it has gone wrong for *you*?

It can be hard to tell if your excess weight is mostly water, since water is everywhere in the body. Even your doctor will have difficulty confirming whether you are retaining fluid. Doctors can tell if you have the severe form of fluid retention known as oedema by pressing a fingertip into your shinbone. If it leaves a dent, you are definitely retaining a great deal of water. Swollen feet or ankles can also be a sign, since excess fluid tends to collect in the lower half of the body. Sometimes the tummy will be tight and swollen (as in premenstrual fluid retention) or the face puffy. However, you can have fluid retention without exhibiting any of these signs.

On the other hand, rapid weight fluctuations, where you have noticed from time to time that you suddenly weigh several pounds more (or less) than you did twenty-four hours ago are a sure sign of fluid retention; only water can cause such a rapid change in your weight.

Solutions – Do's and Don'ts

Don't be tempted to drink less if you believe that you suffer from fluid retention. You must drink enough to allow your kidneys to flush the daily waste products out of your bloodstream. If not, you will usually find that your fluid retention won't improve – it may even become worse. Your body can retain fluid just to dilute an excess of toxic waste substances, as we shall see in Chapter 6.

The best thing to drink is plain water. The worst drinks are tea, coffee and alcohol, which have a diuretic effect. A diuretic is something which stimulates the body to excrete fluid more rapidly, but in the long term this can actually encourage fluid retention as your body will always try to compensate. For the same reason diuretic medicines and herbal products should be treated with caution.

Alcohol can particularly dehydrate you. It reduces the effectiveness of anti-diuretic hormone (ADH), a hormone which slows down the kidneys' excretion of fluid when your body's fluid levels are getting low. This means that you will go on urinating even when your body fluid levels are already low. Drinking a pint of water before going to bed after you have drunk a lot of alcohol can help to reduce both the dehydration and the hangover which results from it!

As with all health matters, the solution to your fluid retention will depend on the *cause*. For the first time in this book you can read about all the possible causes. Once you know why you have fluid retention you will usually be able to put right the harmful changes in your body which have led to it, using the simple dietary measures described in Chapter 9. Then you will literally be able to urinate away much of your excess body weight, sometimes within just a few days.

Some Facts about Water

Water is the most abundant substance in your body, found inside and around each of your cells and in your bloodstream and vital fluids. Water is vital to your body. In a temperate climate, adults can live for up to ten days without water and children for five days. Because your body could be severely damaged by losing only 10 per cent of its normal water levels, your body tries to keep its water balance as even as possible by making you feel thirsty when it is beginning to get dehydrated. Signs of dehydration include dry skin, sunken eyes, mental confusion and concentrated urine.

What is water used for?

Water is an essential component of all your body's living cells. Also, by being dissolved in water, many important vitamins, minerals and other vital substances, as well as waste products produced by your cells, can be transported to where they are needed in your body, or to sites of processing and excretion. Water also helps to regulate your body temperature by producing sweat when you get too hot. The evaporation of sweat has a cooling effect on your skin.

Other uses of water by your body include the production of saliva, which helps you to chew your food, and of digestive juices. Between 12 and 15 pints (7–8.5 litres) of water a day are extracted from the fluid in your tissues to make these juices. After digestion the water is reabsorbed and returned to your tissues. Contrary to popular belief, you do not need to drink fluid with your meals to 'wash down' your food – it is better if you do not dilute your digestive juices in this way.

Where do you get water from?

Water does not just come from the liquids you drink. Up to 2 pints a day can come from food. Fruit, salads and vegetables may contain up to 95 per cent water. Even meat is about 50 per cent water and fish about 70 per cent after cooking. Bread and cheese contain 35 and 40 per cent water respectively. Try leaving them to dry out and see how much they shrink. Even dried fruit is still 20 per cent water.

More than $\frac{1}{4}$ pint of water every day is actually manufactured by your body. Known as metabolic water, this is a by-product formed when food is converted into energy. Your body produces nearly a tablespoon of water from every 100 Calories of food you consume. This water can even be produced from completely dry food; it has nothing to do with the water content of the food itself.

How much water do you need?

Water is lost from your body in urine, sweat, stools and as water vapour in your breath. Heavy sweating can amount to several pints of water a day. Water losses through your breath probably amount to about half a pint a day under normal circumstances.

Most of your water is lost through urine, and it is essential to drink enough fluid to produce the amount of urine that your kidneys need to flush out toxins and waste products. If your urine looks very concentrated, you are probably not drinking enough.

Scientists estimate that most of us need to drink at least 5–6 pints a day – more if our water losses have been high, for instance if you are breast-feeding, or suffer from heavy periods, or diarrhoea, or tend to sweat heavily. It is advisable to drink this amount of fluid even if your thirst levels don't seem to require it. Thirst sensations only begin once dehydration has started. Elderly people in particular often fail to feel thirsty until they are quite dehydrated.

The best drink of all is plain water. Drink it on its own, or use it to dilute drinks like soup and fruit juice. You don't have to drink them neat. A mixture of sparkling water and fresh fruit juice is much better for you than canned fizzy drinks, which are often high in sodium, sugar and chemicals. It tastes good too. Weak fruit or herb teas, such as rosehip, blackcurrant, fennel or chamomile – preferably without sugar, are also good choices, and can be drunk hot or cold.

Water and false weight loss

Water amounting to several pounds of body weight is also lost in the early stages of a low-calorie diet. You urinate this water away within two days when your body uses up its stored carbohydrate (known as glycogen) which is found in muscles and the liver, and is bound up with three times its weight in water. This effect is responsible for much yo-yo dieting, since slimmers believe that they have lost true body weight when they have not. If you have ever tried a short low-calorie diet you probably know how disappointing it is to regain those lost pounds immediately as soon as you resume a normal calorie intake allowing your carbohydrate stores to fill up again.

CHAPTER

Allergic Fluid Retention: How Your Favourite Foods Could Be Turning You into a Sponge

Marjorie lost nearly 14 lbs in one week

One of the biggest causes of fluid retention is food allergy, a problem which could mean that you start holding on to water like a sponge after eating certain foods. If you eat those foods several times every day, your body will never get the chance to release this excess fluid. This chapter explains what allergies can do and how they develop.

Case Study: Marjorie

Marjorie was a forty-eight-year-old supervisor of a care home for the elderly. Although she ate a strict calorie-controlled diet, and was on her feet from 7 a.m. until 9 p.m. most days of the week, up and down stairs, her weight would not budge from 12 stone (168 lb). Worst of all, it was creeping slowly upwards despite the fact that for the last four years she had eaten little but salad with a small portion of lean grilled meat or fish, and thin wheat crackers.

To find some clues as to what might be causing the problem, I asked Marjorie if she ever suffered from various niggling ailments like lack of energy, premenstrual symptoms, joint pains or headaches. It turned out that her doctor had diagnosed arthritis because she had a constant pain in her knees, made much worse by walking upstairs. She had to take painkillers every day.

When I looked at Marjorie's knees, they appeared quite swollen. I was fairly sure that she did not have arthritis but a food allergy which was swelling her up with fluid and making her knees feel tight and painful. I put Marjorie on the Waterfall Diet.

After a few days, I got an excited phone call. 'I just can't seem to get off the loo,' she told me, 'I've been producing buckets and buckets of urine, and my clothes are so loose they're hanging off me!' Marjorie lost nearly 14 lb in that first week. Two weeks later, when she saw me again, she was ecstatic. 'I've been constantly on the loo again and have lost another 7 lb. My knee pains have completely gone, and I'm feeling so full of energy for the first time in years that I'm going to start an exercise class next week!'

Marjorie lost a total of 22 lb on Phase I of the Waterfall Diet, and to tell the truth it was extremely hard for me to get her off it. She was buying new clothes since her old ones didn't fit her any more, toning up her body with exercises, and starting to take care of her appearance again. Within a few months she was looking ten years younger.

Food Allergy and Leaky Gut Questionnaire

• Does your weight sometimes go up or down by 2 lb or more in a single day?

• Has your doctor ever diagnosed you as allergic, even when you were a baby?

• Do you suffer regularly from headaches or migraine?

• Do your fingers or knees regularly feel puffy or painful?

• Do you feel slightly congested in your nose or sinuses a lot of the time, or suffer from asthma or hay fever or a lot of mucus?

• Do you regularly suffer from bloating and flatulence (especially after eating) or diarrhoea?

• Do you sometimes suffer from eczema or other skin rashes?

• Have you ever been diagnosed with irritable bowel syndrome?

If you have answered yes to two or more or of these questions, there is a strong likelihood that you are a food allergy sufferer. If you have answered yes to question 1, your weight problem is probably due to allergic fluid retention.

How Can Ordinary Foods Make You Retain Fluid?

As yet, most doctors are reluctant to believe that food often affects people in this way, but some medical researchers have made a special study of it. One French kidney specialist, Dr G. Lagrue from the Henri Mondor Hospital in Créteil, France, has observed that quite frequently a straightforward case of food allergy is mistaken for the serious kidney condition known as nephrotic syndrome, which results in severe fluid retention due to kidney failure. It appears from his research that some people can react so badly to certain foods that their kidneys behave as if they have this disease.

Patients whom Dr Lagrue has encountered with this kind of food sensitivity have recovered from what was originally diagnosed as nephrotic syndrome after avoiding various foods: cow's milk, pork, wheat, beef and egg. He has found that most of these patients are allergic to several foods, and that the problem foods vary from person to person.

It looks very much as though Marjorie's fluid retention, and that of people similar to her, was a very mild form of the type of allergy that Dr Lagrue describes. In her case, the problem foods turned out to be wheat and yeast. These foods were sending Marjorie's body systems haywire and hindering her blood vessels and kidneys from doing their normal job of siphoning off excess fluid from her tissues.

Fluid retention is probably the most common symptom of food allergy that I have come across in my work as a nutritional therapist.

What Causes Food Allergies?

In Marjorie's case, her problems only started when she was in her forties. She had never had much of a weight problem until then, no pains in her knees, and no fatigue. A lot of people have told me they don't understand how a food allergy (or intolerance as it is more correctly termed) can start apparently out of the blue like this, but the explanation is straightforward. Most experts in food intolerance are now agreed that it is caused by a damaged intestine leaking undigested food particles into the bloodstream. The particles – which should not be in your blood – set off immune system reactions which subsequently cause your symptoms. The kind of damage which leads to this problem is caused by constant irritation of the intestinal (gut) lining.

The vicious circle of intestinal irritation

What can cause irritation to your intestines? As we grow older our digestive juices tend to get weaker. In particular our stomachs can become much less efficient at producing acid – in fact, up to 40 per cent of elderly people are thought to have insufficient stomach acid when digesting a meal. Since good acidity levels are needed to start off the rest of the digestive process, it is easy to see how some people could end up with quite a lot of partly undigested food in their lower intestines, where it can cause irritation and inflammation. You can't necessarily see the undigested particles in your stools. Digestion has to be very poor indeed before your stools start to look abnormal.

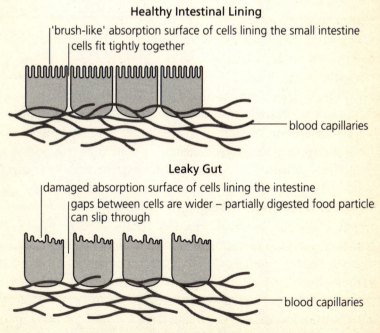

Healthy Intestinal Lining

'brush-like' absorption surface of cells lining the small intestine
cells fit tightly together

blood capillaries

Leaky Gut

damaged absorption surface of cells lining the intestine
gaps between cells are wider – partially digested food particle can slip through

blood capillaries

How the intestinal lining becomes 'leaky'

Your body cannot use food until it has been reduced to its smallest possible particles, known as sugars, amino acids and fatty acids. The lining of your intestine, which normally allows only these items, water and other desirable substances to pass through it into your bloodstream, should be impermeable to undigested food and other potentially harmful substances. But constant irritation can make it too porous, so it starts to leak bacterial toxins and undigested food particles into your bloodstream.

Here your immune system locks on to the particles and treats them like 'foreign invaders'. So food allergy symptoms can be very similar to those caused when your immune system is attacking invading bacteria:

- rashes
- swellings
- joint pains
- headaches
- mucus
- stuffy nose
- fatigue
- flu-like sensations
- diarrhoea

If you suffer from allergy-related fluid retention you will probably, like Marjorie, have one or more of these other symptoms too.

Some people only become allergic to a food after a period of great stress in their lives. Stress can play havoc with your digestion, and so the vicious circle begins: poor digestion → gut irritation and damage → leaky gut, immune system reactions → allergic symptoms and fluid retention. See the panel on pp. 17–19 for more detailed information. It is a vicious circle because, if your gut becomes damaged, its delicate mechanisms for absorbing properly digested food can also start to malfunction. Mild nutritional deficiencies can develop as some of your food passes straight through you without being absorbed. And partially undigested or unabsorbed carbohydrates can be seized by hungry fungi and acid-producing bacteria which reside in the lower part of your gut. If consistently fed too well in this way, they can thrive out of control and gradually extend upwards, colonizing your small intestine. Their presence there causes even more irritation.

Everyday foods

If you have a food intolerance, this will probably involve a food which you eat very often, such as wheat (from bread, pasta, flour, cakes, biscuits and so on), eggs or dairy produce. Most nutritional therapy experts believe that we are more likely to become sensitive to the foods which we eat most often – our immune system simply becomes more reactive to them. If you are allergic to shellfish, for instance, you would usually know it because most people do not eat shellfish every day – it is easy to associate the symptoms with the food. But if you are allergic to a food that you do eat every day, perhaps only in tiny amounts like egg in a cake or a pudding or as a glazing for pastry, your symptoms will either be present more or less all the time, or will come and go at random, never allowing you the chance to make the association.

One woman I treated suffered from migraine only when she was under stress. Yet once she was on the Waterfall Diet she never got migraine again, even when she was under a great deal of stress. Phases I and II of the diet had shown up an allergy to milk and other dairy products, and by steering clear of these foods she was able to remain symptom-free.

Multiple allergies

Sometimes an allergy sufferer will eventually start reacting to many different foods. This is known as multiple allergy syndrome, and is a sign of considerable damage to the intestinal lining and probably also to the liver's efficiency. The damaged intestinal lining will be allowing many toxins, such as those produced by bacteria in the intestines, into the bloodstream. The liver, which has to process toxins, then has a greatly increased workload, and its detoxification enzymes can become overloaded. When this happens, the allergy sufferer can start to feel unwell not just after eating, but after breathing fumes such as vehicle exhaust fumes or artificial perfumes and air fresheners.

Dr Lagrue reports that most of his patients suffering from allergy-related kidney malfunction and the resulting severe fluid retention have multiple allergies, including both foods and fumes.

Antibiotics

The acid-producing bacteria mentioned above are greatly encouraged in people who have taken antibiotics. Your intestines provide a home to many species of bacteria and yeasts/fungi. Some produce a lot of potentially irritating toxins and acids, and are normally kept under control by the other, more 'friendly' bacteria such as *Acidophilus* (as found in yoghurt). But when you take antibiotics, the friendly bacteria are killed and can no longer do this job. They do eventually re-establish themselves, but if you have been on long-term antibiotics, or have been treated regularly with antibiotics for a very long time, your intestines may become colonized by fungi and antibiotic-resistant bacteria, which are very difficult to eradicate. Yeast/fungus type organisms (such as *Candida albicans* or saccharomyces) are unaffected by antibiotics.

The following type of case is very common, and if it sounds like you, you might, in addition to the Waterfall Diet, be in need of treatment to help re-establish your friendly gut bacteria. This would help to heal your leaky gut and prevent you from developing more allergies.

Phase I of the Waterfall Diet is designed to cut out all the foods most likely to be giving you allergic fluid retention. If you lose a lot of weight very quickly during Phase I, it is very likely that your problem is allergy-related. Phase II allows you to test yourself for food allergies so that you will know which foods bring on your problem and can avoid those foods when you move on to Phase III. To receive treatment for a leaky gut, you will need to consult a nutritional therapist (see Useful Addresses on p. 202).

Case Study: John

John suffered badly from acne, and eventually his doctor prescribed antibiotic treatment which lasted about six months. After two months John noticed that he suffered more from intestinal gas and occasional bloating than he used to, but thought little about it. These, however, were signs that his intestines were not absorbing food properly and were become irritated and inflamed.

After a year John was beginning to develop sinus problems, and often seemed to have a stuffy nose and excess mucus. He felt bloated most of the time. He was also finding it hard to get up in the mornings – a problem he had never experienced before. He would sometimes fall asleep in the afternoon at weekends. Although only thirty-five, John put it down to simply getting older. He did not worry much until he found himself usually sleeping ten hours a night and still waking unrefreshed. When his doctor told him there was 'nothing wrong with him', John consulted an alternative doctor who specialized in chronic fatigue syndrome.

The new doctor had his urine tested and found large amounts of a substance that only occurs in the human body when it has a fungus infection in the intestines. John was put on a special diet plus herbs and supplements to control the fungus and help heal his intestinal wall. John quickly lost his sinus problem, which only occurred when he ate dairy produce, and over the next six months he gradually regained his energy levels. His tiredness had been caused by toxins from the fungus leaking from his gut into his bloodstream.

The Chemistry of Allergies

Doctors who specialize in nutritional therapy believe that up to one-third of the Western population suffers from food allergy – the developing of symptoms after consuming certain foods. Symptoms are related not to the substance eaten, but to our reaction to it. So any food can cause any of a hundred symptoms. Wheat might cause headaches or irritable bowel syndrome for some people; dairy produce or eggs could produce them in others, or could give rise to skin rashes or asthma attacks instead. There are two types of allergy: classical allergy, and intolerance or sensitivity reactions.

Classical allergy This type shows symptoms rapidly, and usually produces inflammation of the skin when it is pricked with the offending substance (this is known as a skin prick test). Hay fever, coeliac disease (which results in diarrhoea after eating flour or cereals) and asthma attacks induced by contact with animal fur or house dust mites are all classical allergies. Anaphylactic shock, where the blood pressure falls to life-threateningly low levels, is also a classical allergic reaction, and can cause death. When people die after eating peanuts, for example, it is as a result of anaphylactic shock.

Intolerance or sensitivity reaction Symptoms here are often delayed, intermittent or chronic, and although they may involve the release of histamine by the mast cells of the immune system, a skin prick test may not result in inflammation because they involve a different type of antibody from the classical allergy reaction. Symptoms include migraine, irritable bowel syndrome, joint pains, chronic fatigue and fluid retention.

As explained on p. 13, food intolerance reactions are thought to be due to a combination of incomplete digestion and a leaky gut (intestinal lining). When partially digested proteins, known as peptides, escape through the leaky gut into the bloodstream the immune system responds by attaching IgG antibodies to them. When these peptide/antibody complexes come into contact with histamine-producing white blood cells they stimulate them to release histamine.

Histamine and fluid retention Histamine is a chemical responsible for the physical symptoms experienced by allergy sufferers, including fluid retention. If you have ever suffered from hay fever or insect bites, you will be familiar with some of its effects. Histamine dilates your blood capillaries, producing symptoms such as skin redness, swelling and irritation, and can also constrict the bronchi of the lungs, causing asthma. Capillaries affected by histamine become leaky, and more fluid passes into the surrounding tissues in order that more white blood cells can be carried to the sites where the body thinks the invader is present. If this whole process takes place several times every day, the tissues may not have a chance to release this fluid. Sometimes a few hours' fasting (e.g. overnight) may result in fluid loss, so if you find that you have to get up most nights to urinate, and that you weigh less in the morning, this could be the cause!

Allergy testing If a doctor suspects the presence of an allergy, he/she will normally use skin prick tests and patch tests, where the test substance is placed in contact with your skin. These tests are good for substances like pollen which would normally react with your skin or nasal passages, but are not reliable for food intolerances.

Commercial laboratories sometimes offer blood tests, in which allergies are identified by seeing how your blood cells react when brought into contact with certain foods. This is also an unreliable method since in your body food should never come into contact with your blood.

The Waterfall Diet provides a highly accurate testing method for food intolerances; in technical jargon, it is known as the 'avoidance and challenge' method. More than 90 per cent of food allergy sufferers will be able to identify their problem foods if they follow the instructions carefully.

If you believe you have multiple allergies, you should consult a nutritional therapist or a doctor specializing in nutritional therapy (see Useful Addresses on p. 202). These specialists will help you to improve your digestive ability, reduce the irritation to your intestines that is making them leaky, and repair the damage caused by the irritation.

CHAPTER

Protein Helps You Release Excess Fluid. Are You Getting Enough?

Lesley only lost weight by eating more calories

A lack of protein in your diet can cause fluid retention. We have all seen pictures of third world children with big bellies swollen by fluid retention, and matchstick arms and legs. The technical name for their condition is 'protein-energy malnutrition' and means that they are not consuming enough protein or enough calorie-rich foods in general. The lack of protein in these children's diets prevents their liver from making enough of a substance called albumin, which is essential to prevent fluid retention.

It seems impossible that in the affluent West anyone could suffer from a protein deficiency. In fact most books on nutrition warn us that we are probably eating too much protein and should concentrate more on fruit and vegetables. But some people take this too literally.

Case Study: Lesley

Lesley, a young advertising trainee working in London, had been fighting a weight problem since her teens. Although then she was no more than about a stone (14 lbs) overweight, she felt fat and ugly, especially on the sports field, where she really wanted to shine but had little confidence due to her weight. At fifteen, after trying various diets without much success, she managed with a great effort of willpower to lose 18 lbs by following a diet of just fruit and vegetables and a little dry toast. Soon afterwards she decided to stay on a vegan diet, free of all animal products, because she did not miss meat and dairy produce and felt that this kind of diet was kinder to animals.

Lesley felt great with her new figure and, having lost so much weight, she felt that she could relax her calorie intake, and began eating chocolate, chips and other sugary, fatty foods again. But once she started she could not stop, and the weight problem came back with a vengeance. By seventeen, Lesley weighed more than ever. She was a typical 'yo-yo' dieter, alternating between starving herself for a few weeks and then bingeing on chocolate when the weight had come down a few pounds.

Finally, the scales refused to budge any further, even when Lesley was eating well under 1000 calories a day. When she consulted me, the first thing I noticed was how low in protein her diet was. She ate no breakfast. Her lunch consisted of salad without dressing, and her dinner of plain steamed vegetables and a thin slice of dry wholemeal toast. Lesley ate nothing else at all. No yoghurt, no soya products, no beans, lentils or nuts – the protein-rich foods which her body so badly needed.

After some persuading, because Lesley was afraid to eat extra calories, I put her on the Waterfall Diet. Within two weeks she had lost 4 lbs in spite of eating *more* food than before. Her weight slowly continued towards normal on the diet, and with its help she was able to eat enough protein while remaining vegan.

Protein Deficiency Questionnaire

• Do you regularly avoid eating meat, dairy products or eggs?
• Do you often miss proper meals and snack instead on chocolate, crisps or chips (french fries)?
• Do you often eat meals consisting of just salad vegetables or fruit and vegetables?
• If you are a vegan, do you replace animal products by eating dishes combining rice with soya, beans, lentils or nuts less than once a day?
• Have you eaten less than 1000 Calories a day for more than a few months?

If you answer yes to two or more of the previous questions, there is a possibility that your fluid retention may be partially due to protein deficiency.

How Does a Lack of Protein Cause Fluid Retention?

After a protein-rich meal, your liver uses amino acids to make a type of protein called albumin, which it sends to your bloodstream. Albumin continues to circulate in your blood until it is gradually broken down. Water in the tissues of your body is attracted into your capillaries (your body's smallest blood vessels) by the presence of albumin, and albumin prevents water from leaking out of your capillaries into your tissues. So, without adequate albumin, fluid accumulates in your tissues.

And not eating enough protein can make you gain weight in another way, too. Protein is needed to make hormones, such as the thyroid hormone which helps to keep your metabolism ticking over. One of the first signs of thyroid hormone deficiency can be weight gain as your metabolism slows down.

Other Effects of Protein Deficiency

The most severe form of protein deficiency (mainly seen in the third world) is known as kwashiorkor. It is particularly serious in children since it retards their growth. Apart from fluid retention, other protein deficiency effects include impairment of digestion, muscle wasting and anaemia, because protein is needed to make digestive enzymes, without which your body cannot absorb the food you consume. So to get the amino acids it needs to make vital hormones and enzymes, your body will start to break down its own lean tissue. This is what causes wasting of the arms and legs, while the tummy may look large if it is swollen with fluid retention.

Balance is Essential

Despite the emphasis on protein in this chapter, it is not a good idea to eat *only* protein in an effort to lose weight more quickly. Too much protein would not only dehydrate you but damage your kidneys. Since you need well-functioning kidneys in order to rid you of any fluid you are retaining, you should do everything you can to keep them happy and healthy. Always balance protein with vegetables, grains and other dietary essentials (see Chapter 9).

Case Study: Susan

A protein deficiency can also be caused by eating a very low-calorie diet, even if it seems to contain enough protein. Forty-eight-year-old Susan weighed 11 stone (154 lb), and for five years had been trying to lose weight with the following punishing regime.

She got up at six every morning to jog for half an hour before leaving for work. She went without breakfast and without lunch. In the evening, she told me, she usually ate a salad with a tinned sardine or pilchard and a teaspoon of sunflower seeds. She never ate sugar, butter or other fats or oils, and drank only tea with milk.

Susan also had a number of troubling symptoms, including severely flaking fingernails, reduced sex drive, and increasing tiredness.

Susan was simply not eating enough food to keep her metabolism working properly. Grown women need about $1\frac{1}{2}$ oz of protein a day, which was not being supplied by her daily single sardine.

Susan was another person terrified of eating more calories. The advice I was giving her conflicted with that of every other slimming expert she had ever consulted. It was fortunate that, when I put her on the Waterfall Diet and made her promise to eat three meals a day, she lost several pounds almost immediately.

Working with Susan was very rewarding. After two months she was eating twice as much, weighing 7 lbs less, and feeling much more energetic. Her husband was also extremely pleased: she confessed that her sex drive had returned – something she had never expected to happen. I discharged her from my care when she was ready to start Phase III of the diet, and we both fully expected her weight loss to continue.

Some Facts about Protein

What is Protein? Protein is the material which most of your body is made from: muscle, hormones, enzymes, skin, hair, organs and the fabric of your bones to which calcium clings – all are different types of protein. When you eat protein it is digested into its smallest units, amino acids, which are then absorbed into your bloodstream and help you grow (if you are a child) or repair tissue and make hormones, enzymes and other important substances. If necessary, amino acids can also be converted into energy.

Which foods are rich in protein? High-protein foods include meat, fish, eggs, milk, yoghurt, cheese, soya products, pulses (lentils and beans) and nuts. Rice and other grains are also useful sources of amino acids, but the protein of plants is often called 'incomplete' because it is low in some of the essential amino acids. For example, grains and seeds are low in lysine, whilst pulses and soya products are low in methionine.

Vegetarians and vegans By eating a *variety* of plant proteins, we can still get all the amino acids we need without having to resort to eating animal products like meat and cheese. For example, the lysine lacking in rice can be made up for by eating rice with lentils or with other pulses, since these are rich in lysine. According to the American Dietetic Association, it is probably not necessary to eat them at the same meal. Rice is an ideal accompaniment to beans and lentils, since unlike most other plant foods it is rich in the essential amino acid methionine.

As you can see, you need not develop a protein deficiency if you are vegetarian or vegan (vegans abstain completely from eggs, dairy produce and fish as well as meat). In fact it is generally considered that vegetarians are more healthy than the rest of the population.

How much protein do we need? Children need more protein than adults. But after the age of nineteen your protein need stops increasing and remains about 2 oz (55 g) a day

Protein content of some popular high-protein foods

Food	Protein Content
1 chicken leg without skin	26 g
Batter-fried cod portion 4 oz (110 grams)	20 g
1 large egg, raw or boiled	6 g
Cheddar cheese 1 oz (28 g)	7 g
Oil-roasted, salted peanuts $3\frac{1}{2}$ oz (100 g)	26 g
Rice, cooked $3\frac{1}{2}$ oz (100 g)	3 g
Tofu $3\frac{1}{2}$ oz (100 g)	8 g
Unsalted, dry, roasted cashew nuts $3\frac{1}{2}$ oz (100 g)	15 g
Yoghurt, plain low-fat $3\frac{1}{2}$ oz (100 g)	7 g

for a medium-sized man, and $1\frac{1}{2}$ oz (45 g) a day for a medium-sized woman.

Protein deficiency and fasting Protein deficiency also results from simply not eating, as in the case of starvation, anorexia nervosa or long-term fasting for religious or therapeutic purposes. Your body will begin to break down its own lean tissue to get the amino acids it needs, and will also slow down its metabolism to minimize its protein needs and muscle breakdown. Some researchers report that the metabolism can slow down by as much as 45 per cent. It is not known how long the body takes to return to a normal rate of metabolism or whether it ever does so completely. Severe dieting can also slow down your metabolism. If carried out repeatedly, 'yo-yo' dieting, can have a cumulative effect on your ability to use calories, so that eventually you could start to gain weight on a calorie intake that never caused you problems before.

CHAPTER

Your Personal Waterfall: Making Your Kidneys Work for You

Rarely do we get any nutritional advice for the benefit of our kidneys.

Your kidneys are the most important organ for controlling your fluid balance. If you had no kidneys, all the fluid you drink would accumulate in your blood and around your body's cells, and all the waste products normally excreted by your kidneys would stay inside you and poison you. You would become very ill and soon die.

Kidney stress over many years can lead to kidney damage and to a consequent reduction of their ability to siphon excess fluid out of your body. As we shall see, the major causes of kidney stress include eating too much salt, sugar, protein or fat, and deficiencies of vitamin B6 and the minerals magnesium and selenium. Mercury (as found in tooth fillings) and other toxic substances can also harm your kidneys. This chapter looks at what your kidneys need from you to help them remain as stress-free as possible: the Waterfall Diet is ideal for this.

Case Study: Sally

Sally was not overweight, but had been diagnosed with an illness known as psoriatic arthritis. This is a combination of painful joints (in Sally's case mainly her fingers) and the skin disease known as psoriasis. Since painful joints are often caused by fluid retention, I put her on the Waterfall Diet to see what would happen.

I was really expecting Sally's condition to improve, but two weeks later, her joint pains were as bad as ever. Then I discovered that she had been unwittingly cheating. While the diet forbade salt, I had forgotten to tell her that she must not eat smoked fish, and kippers – foods with a high salt content. Sally had been eating these every day, complaining that otherwise her meals were too bland. It turned out that she loved salt and had always sprinkled her food liberally even when it was already salted. Unsalted food would get a double helping.

Sally spent a very unhappy few days eating food which she did not much enjoy at all, but she soon gained the tremendous benefit of pain-free fingers. Such early relief gave her the incentive to persevere. She also lost 3 lb in weight very quickly, which, as her calorie consumption was not much less than usual, could only be explained by the reduction in her salt intake. As we shall see, salt plays a key role in your fluid balance because it dictates how your kidneys behave. The salt in Sally's diet was interfering with her kidneys, and the resulting fluid retention was making her fingers hurt.

Answer the following questionnaire to see if your fluid retention could be related to kidney stress.

Kidney Function Questionnaire

• Do your ankles regularly swell, especially after you have drunk a lot?
• Do you put two or more spoonsful of sugar in your tea or coffee?
• Do you consume cola, lemonade, sugared commercial 'fruit drinks', milk shakes or other sugary drinks every day?
• Do you eat sweets, chocolate, ice-cream or other sugary items several times every day?
• Do you normally consume bread, pastry, cakes, biscuits and pasta made from white flour?
• Do you regularly eat more than 12 oz a day of high-protein foods such as meat, fish, poultry or cheese?
• Do you eat a lot of fried or greasy food or burgers?
• Do you usually eat highly salted food or add a lot of salt to your food?
• Do you usually eat fresh vegetables or salad vegetables less than once a day?

- Are you vegetarian or vegan?
- Do you have a lot of silver (amalgam) tooth fillings?
- Do you have bowel motions less than once a day?
- Have you ever been diagnosed with a kidney problem?

If you have answered yes to the first question, there is a possibility that your fluid retention may be partially due to kidney stress. If you have answered yes to any of the other questions, this may help you to pinpoint what might be causing the stress to your kidneys.

How Your Kidneys Work

All the blood in your body passes through your kidneys about twenty times an hour. Your kidneys' job is to filter your blood, removing excess fluid and the waste substances dissolved in it and sending it to your bladder from where it is eventually released as urine. Normally the more fluid you drink, the more urine your kidneys will produce for you to excrete. If your fluid intake drops, your kidneys will produce less urine.

Your kidneys lie just above your waist on either side of your spine and under the muscles of your back. Kidneys are delicate and therefore protected by a cushion of fat. Each kidney consists of about 1.25 million nephrons, tiny units which comprise a filtering apparatus (glomerulus) and a long tubule. The glomerulus is actually a dense clump of blood capillaries with a funnel-like structure around it. Fluid and dissolved substances drip out of the porous walls of these capillaries and are collected by the funnel. The fluid drains down through the neck of the funnel into the tubule, which eventually links up with other tubules, all carrying the fluid (now known as urine) towards a larger duct known as the ureter. From the ureter the fluid passes to the bladder.

Under normal circumstances, the glomeruli filter about 48 gallons (180 litres) of fluid from your blood every day, but of course you do not excrete that much urine. The reason is that certain hormones tell your kidneys how much fluid must be reab-

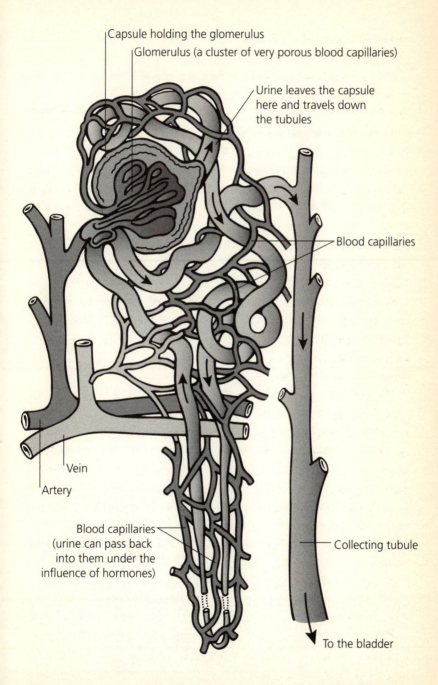

Capsule holding the glomerulus

Glomerulus (a cluster of very porous blood capillaries)

Urine leaves the capsule here and travels down the tubules

Blood capillaries

Vein

Artery

Blood capillaries (urine can pass back into them under the influence of hormones)

Collecting tubule

To the bladder

The nephron: your kidney consists of more than a million of these

sorbed by the tubules and sent back to the blood capillaries surrounding them before your urine reaches the main collecting ducts. If it were not for these hormones, all the fluid in your body would be urinated away within thirty minutes!

Anti-diuretic hormone (ADH)

ADH is secreted by the hypothalamus gland in your head and is stored in your pituitary gland. When ADH levels are low in your blood, the kidney tubules allow little or no water to filter back into your capillaries and the fluid continues to flow down the tubule towards your bladder. But when ADH is present the tubules allow water to filter through their walls and back into your capillaries instead of going to your bladder. ADH therefore reduces the amount of fluid excreted by your kidneys. Its name should help you to remember what effect it has, since 'diuretic' means encouraging the excretion of urine. So 'anti-diuretic' means having the opposite effect.

Aldosterone

While fluid in the tubules cannot get back into your capillaries unless the tubules are made permeable by ADH, most of the fluid would just continue travelling down the tubules were it not for another hormone. Aldosterone is made by the adrenal glands, situated on top of your kidneys. It stimulates the tubules to retain some of the sodium in the fluid passing through them, and the sodium is then drawn back into your capillaries. Sodium always pulls water along with it, and provided that ADH has prepared your tubules by making them porous, water will be reabsorbed before it reaches your bladder. The actual amount reabsorbed depends on how much sodium is retained.

The rule that water follows sodium applies in more ways than one. Consuming too much sodium, in the form of table salt, or as additives (such as monosodium glutamate) in soft drinks and processed foods, forces your body to crave more and more fluid. Just as in Sally's case, your body will retain this fluid until it has the chance to excrete the excess sodium.

Doctors treat fluid retention by prescribing drugs which will stop the kidney tubules from reabsorbing sodium. If less sodium is reabsorbed then less water will be reabsorbed, and so more water will be excreted. These drugs, known as diuretics, have a number of side-effects. In preventing sodium reabsorption, many of them will also prevent the reabsorption of other essential minerals such as potassium and magnesium, leading to inadequate levels of these nutrients. Physical side-effects include dry mouth and rashes, and the drugs can also lead to kidney damage and to a worsening of any pre-existing diabetes or gout.

Drastically reducing your salt intake can help you to avoid or reduce diuretic drugs – with your doctor's permission, of course. If you are already taking these drugs, whether or not you can safely come off them depends on why your doctor has prescribed them. If your fluid retention is due to congestive heart failure, for instance, you will probably need to stay on them to prevent fluid building up in your lungs.

ANH and dopamine

There are two more main hormones involved in kidney function. One, relatively newly discovered, is known as atrial natriuretic hormone (ANH). Secreted by the heart, it has the opposite effect of aldosterone and prevents your tubules from returning sodium to your bloodstream. ANH therefore encourages water excretion. The other, dopamine, has only recently been discovered to have an effect on fluid balance. It too promotes sodium loss in the urine, thus encouraging fluid excretion.

Water excretion by your kidneys is constantly being adjusted by the interplay of all these natural hormones.

Fluid Retention and Minerals

As you can see, sodium plays a vital role in how your body fluid behaves. Your kidneys filter sodium out of your blood, and then return to your blood just the amount which your body needs. When your blood sodium rises, as when you eat salted foods, thirst makes you drink so that the sodium in your blood will not be too concentrated. Then your kidneys excrete the extra water and the extra sodium together.

Why do your kidneys exert such careful control over sodium? The answer is in the job which sodium and other minerals have to do. Two-thirds of your body's fluid has to reside inside your cells, and one-third outside. If this balance is disrupted then your cells could rupture due to the entry of too much water. Alternatively they would collapse if they do not get enough water. Levels of sodium and other minerals control this water balance: if the mineral concentrations inside and outside your cells are correct, the proportions of water attracted to them should also be correct.

It is the tiny electrical charges formed when mineral salts dissolve in water, which are responsible for the minerals attracting water, and which determine whether the minerals end up inside or outside your cells. When minerals are dissolved in water they separate into positively charged sodium particles (ions) and negatively charged chloride particles, and the resulting fluid can conduct electricity. This ability is important for all cells, but especially for nerve cells, which depend on electrical charges to carry messages to your brain, spinal cord and muscles. Those minerals which play an important role due to their ability to carry electrical charges are known as electrolytes.

Your Diet and Your Kidneys

We have all heard about the foods we should or should not eat to help prevent clogged arteries which could lead to a heart attack,

---

The Kidneys' Tasks

- Maintaining water balance
- Excreting toxins and waste products
- Regulating the levels of chemical substances such as sodium, potassium and chloride
- Regulating blood pressure
- Adjusting the body's acid–alkaline balance by selecting which ions (electrically charged particles) to retain and which to excrete, e.g. excreting hydrogen ions in exchange for sodium ions

---

but rarely do we hear any dietary advice for the benefit of our kidneys. Yet a lot of research has been done into the effects of various foods on the health of our kidneys. Since your kidneys play such a vital role in helping you to excrete excess fluid, you could benefit from paying attention to these research findings if you think you may be suffering from fluid retention.

Cut down on sugar

According to researchers, as a nation one of our most damaging dietary habits from the kidneys' point of view is the amount of sugary foods and drinks we consume. Most of us eat about 2 lb of sugar a week (usually without realizing it) in the form of:

- sweets and chocolate
- sweetened tea and coffee
- soft drinks
- breakfast cereals
- jam, marmalade and honey
- cakes
- biscuits
- ice cream

Not only can sugar encourage sodium retention by the kidneys, which could make you retain fluid, but it also has a directly damaging effect on your kidneys and could in time lead to enlarged kidneys and kidney stones.

Dr N. J. Blacklock from the University Hospital of South Manchester in England is one of the world's top experts on diet and kidney function. In one research study he gave 250 grams (about 8 oz) of sugar a day to a group of volunteers and then measured levels of a chemical known as NAG, which is produced by the body when damage has occurred to the kidney tubules. In every case NAG levels were higher after the sugar was consumed.

Over the years, the damage caused by sugar can build up, making your kidneys less efficient and even enlarging them as they try to compensate for the damage. Once kidney damage becomes extensive, whatever its cause, scar tissue can replace your nephrons – that is, your normal kidney tissue.

While the amount of sugar used in Dr Blacklock's study seems like a lot, remember that the *average* sugar consumption in the UK is just over 4 oz a day. So while a lot of people are consuming less than this, an equally large number are consuming *more*. When I was a child, I could easily get through 8 oz of sweets in a day – that is 8 oz of *pure* sugar! I dread to think what effect this kind of diet is having on some young people's kidneys.

Dr Blacklock is also concerned about the effects of sugar on kidney stone formation. About one-third of the UK population produces very high levels of the hormone insulin when they consume sugar, he says, and this excess of insulin has the effect of increasing the kidneys' excretion of calcium. The calcium can then form hard tiny plugs or 'stones' in the kidney tubules. If the stones grow they can get 'stuck' and cause great pain, especially when they shift with the flow of fluid. The treatment of choice for kidney stones is to help them to pass along the tubules and into the bladder. If this does not work, surgery or ultrasound treatment may be required.

High insulin levels stimulated by sugar consumption also have other harmful effects, including the promotion of sodium retention by the kidneys. As we have already seen, sodium retention leads to fluid retention. Diabetics who have to use insulin injections are also prone to fluid retention for the same reason.

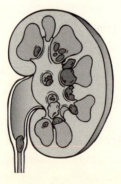

Kidney stones

Vitamin B6, magnesium and other factors

Kidney stones are also encouraged by deficiencies of vitamin B6 and of the mineral magnesium. At least three medical journals, *Urology Research*, the prestigious French journal *Presse Médicale*, and *International Urology and Nephrology*, have published reports that people with a higher intake of these nutrients have a much reduced risk of developing kidney stones, so it really is worth taking good nutrition seriously.

Other dietary factors which researchers have found to impair kidney function include consuming too much protein and fat, and failing to get enough of the trace element selenium in your diet (see below). In 1982 the *British Journal of Urology* reported a study in which 392 kidney stone patients were given a diet high in dietary fibre and low in sugar, white flour and animal protein. Their kidneys began to excrete much lower amounts of calcium, oxalate and uric acid – a clear sign that their risk of developing further kidney stones was now much reduced.

Why dietary fibre? Fibre helps to prevent constipation. As you will see in Chapter 6, constipation can raise the amounts of harmful waste products in your blood and create a much heavier workload for your kidneys. Foods rich in dietary fibre include porridge oats, beans, wholemeal bread and brown rice.

Selenium and your kidneys

One very interesting research study was reported in 1990 in the *Journal of Trace Elements and Electrolytes in Health and Disease*. Eleven healthy volunteers at the Laboratory of Clinical Chemistry in Valeggio, Italy, were given increasing selenium supplements – up to 700 micrograms a day. When the doctors measured how well their kidneys were working compared with before the supplementation, they found that levels of creatinine, a waste substance found in the blood, had dropped by 13 per cent – a very clear indication that the kidneys were working much more efficiently.

Selenium is a trace element which your body requires in tiny amounts: about 75 micrograms a day (one microgram is a thousandth of a milligram, which in turn is one thousandth of a gram). Selenium protects against carcinogenic substances, activates your thyroid hormone and helps you to make an antioxidant enzyme that protects against heart disease. The Italian study seems to be the first to suggest that selenium is also important for kidney function.

In the UK the soil is very poor in selenium, so very little is found in crops. Bread used to make up for this when much of the wheat for flour-making was imported from Canada, a country with selenium-rich soil. But European Union regulations mean that the UK must now use mainly EU wheat, and as a result the nation's average selenium consumption has dropped to about 30 micrograms a day – less than half the recommended necessary intake of 75 micrograms, and below the amount officially designated as adequate for good health.

Another interesting study has been carried out on rats at the Swedish Institute for Genetic and Cellular Toxicology, University of Stockholm. After giving the rats a selenium-deficient diet, Dr U. Olsen and colleagues noticed that the rats' normal kidney function became progressively disturbed.

Another beneficial effect which selenium supplementation may have on your kidneys is to reduce your body's levels of the toxic metal mercury. Dr G. N. Schrauzer's investigation of this use was reported in the German medical journal *Deutsche Zeitschrift für Biologische Zahnmedizin* in 1989. Mercury is found in silver (amalgam) tooth fillings, and over the years is known to leak out in minute amounts into your blood. As your kidneys filter the blood the mercury accumulates in them, gradually causing damage, because it is extremely hard to excrete.

Several medical and dental journals have now reported that the more amalgam fillings there are in the mouth, the more mercury can collect in the kidneys. For instance, researchers at the University of Umea in Sweden have found that mercury levels rose continuously after amalgam fillings were placed for the first time in eight healthy individuals. A study reported in the *Swedish Dental Journal* in 1987 found that when the bodies of twelve people were examined at autopsy, those with amalgam fillings had much higher levels of mercury in their kidneys than those without. Studies carried out on sheep (an animal chosen because it spends much of its time chewing) by Canadian dental researcher Murray Vimy suggest that an average number of amalgam fillings could over a lifetime destroy 50 per cent of your kidney cells.

The good news is that selenium helps you to excrete mercury by binding to it. But to be on the safe side, many people are having their silver fillings gradually replaced with white ones or with inlays. Most fillings eventually need replacing anyway. When silver fillings are removed, ask your dentist to use a rubber dam to prevent you from absorbing any mercury during this process. And do not swallow it.

If kidneys work better with more selenium, it would certainly make sense to start taking supplements since in the UK there seems no other way to increase our selenium intake to the level recommended by the Government. Apart from meat and fish, the only other good natural source is brazil nuts, but you would need to eat between ten and twenty a day to raise your selenium intake from 30 to 75 micrograms. Dr Guidi's Italian patients were presumably eating a diet deficient in selenium, and this is why the supplements helped them. The generally preferred forms of selenium supplementation are selenium-rich yeast, and L-selenomethionine. Supplements of these products are considered perfectly safe at levels of up to 200 micrograms a day. Another supplement which (very slowly) helps to carry excess mercury out of the body is the amino acid n-acetyl cysteine (NAC), also available as supplements.

Do remember, all dentists agree that the best way to avoid fillings is to avoid sugary foods.

Tips for a healthy diet

Don't be surprised if you are starting to feel confused about the 'ideal' diet. As we saw in Chapter 3, too little protein causes fluid retention. Now we find that too much protein stresses the kidneys. Too little fat is bad for you – and too much fat is also bad for you. How can the average person get it right? While most of the dietary advice you will need is in Chapter 9, here are a couple of helpful tips to be going on with:

- The bulk of your food should be minimally processed. That is to say, eat brown rice in preference to white, and wholemeal bread instead of white, nine times out of ten.
- Wherever possible, prepare your food from scratch instead of buying it ready-made. That way you know how much fat and sugar it contains, and you can control your intake of these damaging items more easily.

Medical research is showing again and again that a diet based on the principles of the Waterfall Diet will protect your kidneys from the illnesses and malfunctions that so often come with age and lead to fluid retention. And don't worry if you have been following bad habits up to now; it is never too late to reap the benefits of changing them.

Some Facts about Salt

Only 10 per cent of the salt in our diet comes from the natural salt in foods. The rest comes from adding salt to food. Salt is used both as a condiment in cookery, and as a food additive and preservative.

Foods high in salt include bacon, ham, salami, sausages, pork pies and other preserved meats, canned fish, smoked fish, soy sauce, yeast extract, many cheeses, salted butter, salted peanuts and other packet snacks, packet and canned soups and sauces, most bread, stock cubes and ready-cooked meals for reheating. The regular consumption of these foods, plus the salt added to your food, can easily lead to an intake of 12–17 g a day – the World Health Organization recommends no more than 5g.

The potential damage A high salt intake has been linked with high blood pressure and strokes because it encourages the body to retain water. (It is the extra volume of blood in the arteries caused by this extra fluid that raises the pressure inside them.) However, not all individuals with high blood pressure respond to a low-salt diet – some are thought to be more salt-sensitive than others. Recent research also shows that a high salt intake encourages osteoporosis (brittle bone disease). Salt also seems to increase the lungs' sensitivity to histamine, and studies have shown that asthma is worsened by a high salt intake.

As described by Dr Nadya Coates in her book *A Matter of Life*, sodium chloride, in contact with water, breaks down in your body to hydrochloric acid and sodium hydroxide (caustic soda). The hydrochloric acid is removed from your blood and used in your digestion processes. The sodium hydroxide remains as an irritant to your cells, and has to be neutralized with lactic acid. Severe sodium hydroxide irritation may be experienced as a burning sensation in the affected parts of the body, even though these parts may feel cold to the touch. Some authorities believe that the resultant damage to cells could act as a trigger for cancer.

It's easy to cut down You can reduce your salt intake by avoiding the above-mentioned high-salt foods, by exercising caution with all foods not prepared at home (especially if they taste salty), and by using low-sodium salt or salt substitute (usually potassium chloride) in cooking and at the table.

How's your zinc? Children who are faddy eaters and eat only sweet or highly salted foods may have had their sense of taste damaged by a zinc deficiency. It is quite hard to get substantial amounts of zinc from your diet unless you eat mostly wholefoods, meat and fish; zinc deficiency is therefore becoming increasingly common. To zinc-deficient people, most foods taste too bland unless plenty of salt or other flavouring is added. Once the zinc deficiency has been corrected, your child may begin to enjoy a wider range of foods.

Organic sodium may be good for you Salt (in chemical terms, sodium chloride) is not the only source of sodium in your diet. Most natural foods contain only a small sodium content, but it is probably beneficial. The best sources are fresh fish, meat, eggs, celery, beetroot, carrots, radishes, spinach and watercress. Sodium occurring in such foods is normally found incorporated in plant or animal cells and is therefore in organic form and may be handled differently by the human body when consumed. We should point out that 'organic' is not used here in the usual sense of food grown without pesticides and fertilizers. An organic mineral is one in the form found in living tissues as opposed to the minerals found in rocks, for example.

The organic sodium found in vegetables such as celery may help to keep inorganic sodium (from salt) in solution, thus helping your body to eliminate it.

The Medicines That Can Make You Fat: What Is Your Doctor Prescribing?

Under the law, proof is not required that a medicine be safe, only that its benefits should outweigh its side effects.

Fluid retention can be a side-effect of a surprisingly large number of both necessary and unnecessary prescription medicines, particularly female hormonal treatments, painkillers, steroids and blood pressure medications.

Case Study: Jean

Jean consulted me as a last resort. 'My doctor says I've got to lose weight for my blood pressure', she said 'otherwise my heart could get damaged. He sent me to the dietician, who gave me a 1000-calorie-a-day diet, but I was already eating less than that so I'm gaining weight on it. What can I do? They won't believe me when I tell them how little I'm eating.'

Poor Jean was very distressed. One of the first things I noticed was her swollen ankles, so I immediately suspected that she was retaining fluid. 'How long have they been swollen?' I asked. Jean replied that she had first become aware of them soon after beginning to take the beta-blocker drugs her doctor had given her for her blood pressure. It turned out that the weight gain had also started around this time. I asked Jean some more questions designed to find out if she was an allergic type or possibly deficient in protein, but the drugs remained the only clue to her problem.

Medical reference books confirmed that beta-blockers can indeed cause fluid retention, but Jean's doctor had not put two and two together. Few doctors would have done. Although Jean seemed very nervous of questioning his advice, she promised to get up the courage to return, show him her swollen ankles, and discuss the possibility that her weight gain might be due to the medication.

Answer the following questionnaire to see if prescription medicines could be causing your fluid retention.

Medicines Questionnaire

- Are you taking any of the medicines described in the table below?
- Did the start of your fluid retention/weight gain seem to coincide with beginning to take this medicine?
- Has your fluid retention/weight gain worsened since you started to take this medicine?
- Have you ever taken any of the medicines described as causing possible kidney damage?
- Has your fluid retention/weight gain only become noticeable since the time when you took this drug?

If you believe that a drug may be causing your fluid retention, it is very important that you do not come off it without discussing the problem with your doctor.

Drugs which Can Promote Fluid Retention

Drug Type Generic Name	Some Common Brand Names	Used Mainly for	Effects on Fluid Balance	Possible Alternatives
ACE Inhibitors: e.g. Captopril	Acepril Capoten	High blood pressure and congestive heart failure	Toxic to kidneys. May also cause swellings due to allergic fluid retention.	Nutritional therapy Herbal therapy

Table continued

Drug Type Generic Name	Some Common Brand Names	Used Mainly for	Effects on Fluid Balance	Possible Alternatives
Beta Blockers: e.g. Metoprolol Pindolol Propranolol	Betaloc Lopressor Visken Inderal	High blood pressure, angina, anxiety	May reduce the heart's ability to pump the blood through the kidneys, thus encouraging fluid retention	Nutritional therapy Herbal therapy Relaxation techniques
Calcium Channel Blockers: e.g. Nifedipine	Adalat Adipine Cardilate MR Coracten Unipine XL	Angina, high blood pressure, Raynaud's disease	May reduce the heart's ability to pump the blood through the kidneys, thus encouraging fluid retention	Nutritional therapy Herbal therapy Homoeopathy
Central Alpha Stimulant: Clonidine Methyldopa	Catapres Dixarit Aldomet	High blood pressure, migraine, menopausal hot flushes	Can cause sodium retention and consequent fluid retention	Nutritional therapy Herbal therapy Homoeopathy Traditional Chinese medicine
Vasodilators: e.g. Diazoxide Hydralazine Minoxidil	Eudemine Apresoline Loniten Regaine	High blood pressure. Regaine is sometimes used to treat male baldness.	May reduce the heart's ability to pump the blood through the kidneys, thus encouraging fluid retention	Nutritional therapy Herbal therapy
Reserpine	No longer used in the UK	High blood pressure	Can cause sodium retention and consequent fluid retention	Nutritional therapy Herbal therapy

Table continued

Drug Type Generic Name	Some Common Brand Names	Used Mainly for	Effects on Fluid Balance	Possible Alternatives
Loop Diuretics: e.g. Bumetanide Frusemide	Burinex Lasix	Fluid retention	Capable of causing kidney damage. All diuretics can worsen high-protein type fluid retention	While there are several herbal diuretics, these will not solve the underlying problem causing the fluid retention. See Chapter 9 for dealing with the causes
Thiazide Diuretics	Hygroton Saluric	Fluid retention	Capable of causing kidney damage. All diuretics can worsen high-protein type fluid retention	
Potassium-Sparing Diuretics	Dytac Amilamont Amilospare Berkamil	Fluid retention	All diuretics can worsen high-protein type fluid retention	
NSAIDS: e.g. Aceclophenac Acemetacin Aspirin-type painkillers Azapro-pazone Diclofenac sodium Diflunisal Etodolac Fenbufen Fenoprofen Flurbiprofen Ibuprofen Indomethacin Ketoprofen	Preservex Emflex Anadin Nuseals Rheumox Voltarol Diclomax Dolobid Lodine Lederfen Fenopron Froben Ocufen Brufen Nurofen Cuprofen Indocid, Flexin Ketofen Oruvail Orudis	Pain and inflammation	Prevent production of prostaglandins involved in kidney function	Nutritional therapy Herbal therapy Acupuncture Homoeopathy

Table continued

Drug Type Generic Name	Some Common Brand Names	Used Mainly for	Effects on Fluid Balance	Possible Alternatives
Ketorolac	Acular, Toradol			
Mefenamic acid	Ponstan Meflam			
Meloxicam	Mobic			
Nabumetone	Reliflex			
Naproxen	Naprosyn Synflex Naprotec			
Phenyl-butazone	Butacote			
Piroxicam	Feldene			
Sulindac	Clinoril			
Tenoxicam	Mobiflex			
Tiapofenic acid	Surgam			
Tolmetin	Tolectin			
Corticosteroid Drugs: e.g. Beclometha-sone	Becotide Becloforte	Pain and inflammation, asthma	Can cause sodium reten-tion and consequent fluid retention	Nutritional therapy Herbal therapy Acupuncture Homoeopathy
Betamethasone	Betnesol			
Dexametha-sone	Decadron Maxidex			
Fludrocortisone	Florinef			
Flunisolide	Syntaris			
Prednisone } Prednisolone }	Deltacortril Precortisyl Forte			
Triamcinolone	Adcortyl Kenalog Nasocort			
Amphotericin	Fungilin Ambisone Fungizone	Anti-fungal	Toxic to the kidneys	Nutritional therapy
Oestrogen	Premarin Premique Prempak	Contraceptive Pill and HRT	Causes sodium retention and consequent fluid retention	There are many alternative methods of contraception

Table continued

45

Drug Type Generic Name	Some Common Brand Names	Used Mainly for	Effects on Fluid Balance	Possible Alternatives
Progestogen	Duphaston Provera Primolut Cyclogest	Contraceptive Pill and HRT	Causes sodium retention and consequent fluid retention	Nutritional therapy, Herbal therapy, Traditional Chinese medicine and Homoeopathy
Danazol	Danot	Endometriosis	Reasons for fluid retention are unclear	Nutritional therapy Herbal therapy Traditional Chinese medicine Homoeopathy
Phenothiazines	Largactil Stelazine	Mental illness	May reduce the heart's ability to pump the blood through the kidneys, thus encouraging fluid retention.	Nutritional therapy is an effective treatment in those many cases of mental illness caused by abnormally high nutritional needs which have gone unfulfilled
Tricyclic anti-depressants: e.g. Amitryptiline Clomipramine Desipramine Imipramine Nortriptyline	Tryptizol Tryptafen Lentizol Anafranil Pertofran Tofranil Allegron Motipress Motival	Mental illness	Fluid retention may occur as an allergic reaction	Ditto above

Table continued

Drug Type Generic Name	Some Common Brand Names	Used Mainly for	Effects on Fluid Balance	Possible Alternatives
Insulin	Any brand, and also high levels of natural insulin	Diabetes	Can cause sodium retention and consequent fluid retention	Do not attempt to stop insulin treatment. Nutritional therapy can help but should be used under the supervision of a doctor
Metoclopramide	Maxolon Paramax Gastrobid	Nausea, vomiting, migraine	Causes rise in aldosterone (sodium-retention hormone). May also cause swellings due to allergic fluid retention	Alternatives depend on treating the causes of these problems
Cephalosporin antibiotics: e.g. Cephaclor	Distaclor	Bacterial infections	Fluid retention may occur as an allergic reaction	Vitamin C megadoses, raw garlic, herbal anti-bacterials. Use under medical supervision
Co-trimoxazole antibiotics	Septrin	Bacterial infections	Capable of causing kidney damage	Ditto above
Acyclovir anti-virals	Zovirax	Viral infections	Capable of causing kidney damage	Vitamin C megadoses. Uña de gato (cat's claw) herb. Possibly olive leaf extract, though research on humans is lacking

Sources of drug toxicity information: on-line search of drug databases, American Society of Health drug information, British National Formulary

The table contains brand names as well as generic drug names, and is intended for at-a-glance reference. The descriptions in the text on the following pages contain only generic names (so you may not find your particular medication named here) but offer fuller details.

Drugs Used to Reduce High Blood Pressure

As blood is pumped through the arteries, the pressure it exerts against your artery walls is known as your blood pressure. It can be raised above normal by hormonal imbalances, by narrowing of your arteries (which forces your heart to pump harder), by fluid retention and by excessive stickiness (viscosity) of your blood. High blood pressure must be treated. Doctors normally use drugs which:

- act as diuretics, or
- help to keep the arteries as wide (dilated) as possible, or
- prevent your hormones from quickening your heartbeat

Captopril

This is a type of drug known as an ACE inhibitor. It is used to treat high blood pressure and congestive heart failure, (a condition in which the heart's pumping ability begins to fail), and works by blocking the chain of reactions which results in the body's production of aldosterone. As explained in Chapter 4, aldosterone stimulates your kidney tubules to retain some of the sodium in the fluid passing through them. The sodium is then drawn back into your blood capillaries, along with water, increasing the amount of water in your blood and thus the quantity of fluid in your body. By preventing this action, ACE inhibitor drugs reduce fluid. With less blood to pump around the body the heart's workload is reduced, and so is the blood pressure.

Between 4 and 12 per cent of patients who are prescribed this drug find its side-effects too severe to remain on it. It can cause swellings (localized fluid retention) and can be quite toxic to the kidneys; doctors are instructed to monitor their patients' kidney function while they are on it.

Pindolol, propranolol and metoprolol

These drugs are known as beta-blockers. They are used to treat high blood pressure, angina, anxiety and migraine. They work by preventing the body from responding to stress in its usual way. When the stressful emotions (anger, fear, excitement, tension, anxiety and so on) are felt, hormones such as adrenaline are released by the body and stimulate the heart to beat faster and harder. Beta-blockers reduce this stimulation, slowing down the heart and reducing its pumping force, which helps to keep the blood pressure down. In angina sufferers it helps to prevent pain, and in anxiety sufferers it reduces the physical symptoms of anxiety.

Many of the side-effects of beta-blockers are related to the slowing down of the heart: coldness and circulatory problems, depression, impotence and memory loss. Between 6 and 16 per cent of people on pindolol suffer from fluid retention in hands, feet and ankles.

Nifedipine

This is a so-called calcium channel blocker drug, used to treat high blood pressure, angina and the 'cold fingers syndrome' known as Raynaud's disease. The drug decreases the contractions of muscles in arteries and veins by blocking the entry of calcium into cells. This keeps them dilated, which reduces the blood pressure and improves the circulation. Nifedipine is often prescribed together with beta-blockers to counteract some of the circulation problems which these drugs produce.

Drug toxicity researchers are worried at the lack of data on the potential adverse effects of calcium channel blocker drugs. The main side-effect, suffered by 10–30 per cent of patients taking nifedipine on a long-term basis, is fluid retention, especially in the ankles. In addition 25 per cent of patients develop dizziness, lightheadedness, flushing or heat sensation and headaches.

Methyldopa and clonidine

These are another type of drug which reduces blood pressure by dilating the arteries. Acting mainly on blood pressure-controlling sites in the brain, they prevent arteries from contracting in response to nerve stimulation. Clonidine is also used to treat menopausal hot flushes and to prevent migraine. Not used much nowadays, both drugs can cause sodium retention leading to fluid retention.

Diazoxide, hydralazine and minoxidil

Patients with high blood pressure which does not respond to a combination of beta-blocker and diuretic drugs may be given one of these drugs, which act directly on the muscles of the arteries, helping to dilate them. One of their most common side-effects is sodium retention, leading to fluid retention and weight gain. Minoxidil is also used as a scalp application to treat male-pattern baldness.

Reserpine

Derived from the roots of an Indian climbing shrub known as rawolfia, this drug lowers the blood pressure and slows the heart. It has a sedative effect and was formerly used to treat mental illness. Reserpine can also cause sodium retention and consequent fluid retention. It is no longer prescribed in the UK.

Drugs Used to Promote Urination (Diuretics)

As already discussed, fluid retention is one of the factors which promotes high blood pressure. The more fluid the heart has to try to pump around the body, the harder its pumping force and so the greater the pressure exerted on the artery walls. To help reduce this pressure doctors will often prescribe a diuretic drug to prevent the kidney tubules from holding on to sodium and water. More water will then be excreted as urine. As we have already seen, many blood pressure-reducing medications also promote fluid retention, so it is common practice for a doctor to administer a beta-blocker and a diuretic together.

Diuretic drugs are also used to treat fluid retention caused by kidney or liver disease and congestive heart failure. As less blood is pumped through the kidneys, the body starts to retain more and more fluid. If these fluid levels rise too high there is a risk of the body becoming starved of oxygen, so it is essential to reduce them. Doctors do this by administering diuretic drugs.

There are three types of diuretic drugs: loop diuretics, thiazides and potassium-sparing diuretics.

Loop diuretics: bumetanide and frusemide

These drugs are known as loop diuretics because they inhibit sodium reabsorption in a particular section of the kidney tubule known as the loop of Henle. They are very powerful and are known to inhibit the body's reabsorption of potassium, magnesium and calcium, which could cause deficiencies of these important substances.

Although this is not among the most frequent side-effects of bumetanide and frusemide, both drugs are capable of causing kidney damage. Like all diuretics they could worsen high-protein type fluid retention (see p. 98).

Thiazide diuretics

Thiazides comprise the largest group of diuretic drugs, and are moderate in potency. Like the loop diuretics they deplete the body of sodium, magnesium and potassium, and may raise uric acid levels in the blood. They are also capable of causing kidney damage. Like all diuretics they could worsen high-protein type fluid retention (see p. 98).

Potassium-sparing diuretics: spironolactone, triamterine and amiloride

This group is so-called because the drugs it comprises are thought not to result in such large potassium losses from the body as the other types of diuretics. Like all diuretics they could worsen high-protein type fluid retention (see p. 98), so should never be prescribed for this type of fluid retention.

Painkillers

Two types of drugs are used to treat pain and inflammation, and are prescribed on a long-term basis in conditions such as rheumatoid arthiritis. The first type are known as non-steroidal, because they are not based on imitations of the body's own steroid hormones; the other type are known as steroidal anti-inflammatory drugs, and are similar to cortisone. It is not widely known that both types of painkillers can promote fluid retention when used long-term.

Non-steroidal anti-inflammatory drugs (NSAIDS)

These drugs have a large number of generic names (see table on pp. 44–5) and treat pain by blocking the body's production of prostaglandins – hormone-like substances which play a part in causing pain sensations. Prostaglandins are also involved in the kidneys' ability to extract fluid from the blood, and the blocking of this ability is one reason why long-term use of these drugs causes fluid retention. Most NSAIDS can also cause some degree of kidney damage when used in high doses regularly on a long-term basis (rather than just for the occasional headache).

Corticosteroid drugs

Again, see the table on p. 45 for generic names. These steroid drugs, which resemble hormones produced by the body's adrenal glands, are given by mouth to treat rheumatoid arthritis, ulcerative colitis and other inflammatory diseases, and asthma, or may be applied externally as creams or ointments to treat skin inflammations such as eczema. Some corticosteroid drugs such as beclomethasone and fluticasone are also available for asthma patients to inhale. These products include Becotide and Flixotide inhalers.

The dangers of steroid drugs are well known, and should not be underestimated. It is especially dangerous to stop taking them suddenly. Regular use of these drugs makes the body stop producing its own corticosteroids and rely on the drugs instead.

Corticosteroids cause fluid retention by encouraging the body to retain sodium. Other side-effects include shrinkage of the adrenal glands, osteoporosis, susceptibility to infections, thrush, diabetes, mental disturbances such as mood swings, thinning of the skin, acne, and the growth of extra body or facial hair.

Anti-Fungal Drugs

Amphotericin

You may be prescribed amphotericin if you suffer from a fungal or yeast infection such as thrush. It is normally prescribed for six to ten weeks and sometimes longer. Fungal infections can develop in your mouth and throat, intestines or vagina. They are more likely to occur if your immune system is depressed through lack of proper nourishment, from taking immune-suppressing drugs such as corticosteroids, or from a life-threatening condition such as AIDS.

Amphotericin is potentially harmful to the liver and kidneys. This is the reason why it is included here among the list of potentially fluid retention-promoting drugs.

Sex Steroids

Oestrogens and progestogens

You may never have heard oestrogens and progestogens (known in the United States as progestins) referred to as steroid drugs before, but this is indeed what they are, and how they are classified in medical books. Steroids are hormones with a particular type of chemical structure, and these female sex hormones conform to that structure.

Synthetic or semi-synthetic ethinyloestradiol, mestranol and progestogen are normally used in the contraceptive pill rather than the natural hormones oestradiol (the most active form of oestrogen) and progesterone. Although real oestrogen (extracted from urine) can be administered as patches for hormone replacement therapy (HRT), it is not usually given by mouth since it is not well absorbed from the intestines. Progesterone cannot be taken by mouth as it is broken down by the digestive processes.

The synthetic forms are far more potent than our own natural hormones. Although they are administered in tiny amounts, their effects on the female body are extremely powerful and they are more difficult to break down and excrete.

Synthetic oestrogens and progestogens both encourage sodium retention and therefore fluid retention. This is a major side-effect of both drugs, and can lead to breast tenderness, tummy swelling and a weight gain of several pounds.

Other Drugs
Further drugs which can cause fluid retention include:

- tricyclic antidepressants and phenothiazines, used to treat mental illness
- the antiviral drug aciclovir
- danazol, a masculinizing drug given for endometriosis
- insulin, which is essential for the treatment of insulin-dependent diabetes
- metoclopramide, used to treat nausea, vomiting and migraine
- some antibiotics, which are occasionally toxic to the kidneys but are more likely to cause fluid retention by provoking an allergic reaction.

It should be remembered that any drug, like any food, can cause allergic symptoms in sensitive individuals, and that allergy can result in considerable fluid retention (see Chapter 2).

Do I Really Need My Drugs?
Only your doctor can answer this question, but not unless you ask. The following questions can help you to make more informed decisions about your treatments.

- Is my problem serious enough to need medical treatment right now?
- Will your treatment cure it or just help me to cope with it?

- Is my problem likely to get worse even if I take your treatment?
- What side-effects does your treatment have?

In case your doctor wishes to shield you from knowing about all the potential side-effects of the recommended medicine (because you might start imagining you develop them!) you should also do your own research to discover the potential side-effects. Your local pharmacist will have a reference book where you can look them up. Other books will be available through your local reference library.

It may be that, although you cannot come off your medication now, you might be able to if you obtain an improvement in your condition by using natural medicine.

Do Alternatives Work as Well as Conventional Medicine?

That depends on what your health problem is and what you are trying to achieve. If all you want is a painkiller for an occasional headache, conventional medicine provides cheap, effective and convenient solutions. But if you have arthritis which is slowly getting worse, or migraine attacks every week, the treatment is still basically only painkillers. With a few notable exceptions such as antibiotics, most medical treatments do nothing to stem the progress of an illness. They only act as palliatives, helping you to cope with it a little more easily provided that you continue taking the medication every day. As soon as you stop taking it, the palliative effect is lost. This means that most medical treatments are not, in fact, effective in achieving what you want – which is presumably to stop or reverse the illness rather than control the symptoms.

Natural medicine, on the other hand, is capable of real cures for chronic illnesses. Nutritional therapy can be especially effective since so much ill health – including most of the health problems named in this chapter – is caused by faulty nutrition and so can be reversed by giving your body what it needs. The principle is the same as when you treat an ailing plant by giving it more minerals, or changing it to a lime-rich soil. The cells in your body have much in common with plants.

Because it is so nourishing, following the Waterfall Diet is likely to bring you more benefits than just reducing fluid retention. You will probably sleep better and have better skin, more energy and fewer headaches. If you are a woman, problems like period pains and PMS can disappear. More serious health problems such as asthma, arthritis and high blood pressure can also improve, although for these you may need a more tailored nutritional treatment, obtainable from a nutritional therapist (see Useful Addresses on p. 202).

If you decide to try a particular natural therapy, do tell your doctor in case there are any objections. If he/she has any worries your natural therapist should be able to supply you with information to reassure him. Not only are therapies like nutritional therapy very well backed up by science, but consumer surveys (for instance the 1995 UK Consumers Association study) carried out on people who have used natural therapies show that the vast majority find them helpful and good value for money. If you or your doctor are interested in nutritional therapy research, see Useful Addresses for more information. Finally, don't allow yourself to feel intimidated by your doctor or to be afraid of getting a second opinion. There is sure to be a doctor in your area who is interested in natural medicine or even employs natural medical practitioners in his/her surgery.

Taking Responsibility For Your Health

In natural medicine, we talk about taking responsibility for your health as the first step in preventing or combating health problems like fluid retention. Taking responsibility for your health means treating your body with respect and understanding that whether it functions well for you or not often depends on how well you obey natural laws which you cannot change. Natural medicine practitioners try to help people understand the limitations of drug-based medicine and particularly its dangers.

Is Bad Health Really Preventable?

Most things become preventable when we understand what causes them and are able to influence those causes. Unfortunately the majority of doctors are poorly informed about nutritional therapy and natural medicine. The medical journals on which they rely play a large part in this. Pick up any of these journals and it is clear that not only is their main content about pharmaceutical drugs but they are also funded by large glossy advertisements from pharmaceutical companies.

While this does not necessarily mean that they cannot deal fairly with types of medicine other than drugs (and surgery) research carried out using natural medicine is often not included. It is almost impossible for practitioners of low-technology medicine to compete with the marketing budgets of the billion pound pharmaceutical industry. As a result most doctors are not as up to date with some of the excellent and effective principles of nutritional therapy as they could be.

More Facts about the Contraceptive Pill and HRT

Oestrogens and progestogens are used in both the contraceptive pill and HRT preparations. Both types of drug are associated with fluid retention.

Other undesirable side-effects At a conference held in London in 1997 by Doctors Against Sex Hormone Abuse (DASH), many of those attending said they were worried

by the growing tendency to prescribe these drugs, partly because of their own experiences. Dr Margaret White described how she found it harder to come off HRT than to stop smoking. Dr Elizabeth Price developed severe side-effects when she used HRT, and had to stop taking it. When she investigated the national statistics, she found that the suicide rate was twice as high in women taking HRT than in others. UK hospital admission rates are much higher among pill users than among those who use other contraception methods.

Most of the side-effects are mood disturbances, including aggression, depression and violence. According to a report by the British Royal College of General Practitioners, neurotic depression is the most common reason for women to come off the Pill. Interactions between hormones and other drugs such as tranquillizers, caffeine and alcohol can make side-effects worse.

Dr Ellen Grant reported that, while it was once thought that only oestrogen increased the risk of thrombosis and heart attacks among Pill users, it is now known that women over thirty-five who smoke and take contraceptives containing progestogens are 400 times more likely to have a heart attack than those who do not take the Pill.

Professor Michael Steel looked at more than 75 studies linking the Pill with breast cancer. Women who start taking the Pill at an early age and continue taking it for a long time are four times more likely to get this disease. Out of every 100 women who use oestrogen-only HRT for ten years, one will develop breast cancer. Out of every 100 women who use combined oestrogen-progesterone HRT for ten years, two will develop it. Professor Steel said that claims that taking the Pill reduces the risk of ovarian cancer by 30–40 per cent do not bear this out.

Professor James Walker reminded the audience that the synthetic oestrogen diethylstilboestrol (DES) was at first marketed as totally safe and given to 4.8 million pregnant women in the USA. Eventually found to be ineffective, it was banned in 1971. Twenty years later, vaginal cancers were being discovered in daughters of the women who took DES. Many progestogens are derivatives of the male hormone testosterone, and can have masculinizing side-effects, he says.

Drug databases also report the following side effects:

- Oestrogen-containing contraceptive pills can cause a

deficiency of the B vitamin folic acid. Folic acid deficiency makes you more prone to heart disease and Alzheimer's disease, and can cause birth defects.

- If you are taking oestrogen and develop sudden severe tummy pain there is a possibility you may have a liver tumour

Taking oestrogen can

- make you more likely to develop vaginal thrush.
- change the surface of your eyes, causing problems with wearing contact lenses.
- cause breast changes, including tenderness and enlargement.
- increase your risk of stroke, heart attack, gall bladder disease, birth defects in your children, disturbances in vision, cancers and high blood pressure.
- cause irregular brown patches to develop on your face within one month to two years. These may be permanent.

Taking progestogens can

- cause bleeding and spotting between periods.

- cause severe depression.
- increase your risk of heart attack, stroke, high blood pressure and embolism of the eyes (eye damage due to small blood clots).
- cause headaches, nervousness, hair loss and changes in sex drive.

Coming off HRT If you are on HRT and decide to stop taking it, do so under your doctor's supervision. Most women find that due to withdrawal symptoms it is best to reduce the HRT dose very gradually over about a year. One good method is to start by taking the patches off your skin for an hour or two each day, gradually building up the amount of time you spend without them. In the meantime following the Waterfall Diet will help your body balance its own hormones, especially if you eat a lot of soya products such as soya milk, tofu and soya flour. In Japan, where women eat soya every day, there is no word for 'hot flushes' because they are so rare!

If you are taking HRT to prevent osteoporosis, you may be interested to know that at least three medical journals have now reported that one of the most effective ways to prevent – and even reverse – osteoporosis is to consume foods and supplements rich in many minerals, especially magnesium and zinc, which are just as important as calcium and even more likely to be depleted in the average diet. Regular exercise like walking, swimming and trampolining is also very effective.

How Polluted Are You? Your Body May Be Using Water to Dilute Toxins

Who says there's no such thing as cellulite?

Two main types of fluid retention can be caused by internal pollution – by the presence in your body of high levels of substances that should not be there. The first type is cellulite, while the second is related to inflammation and leakage of your blood vessels – known in its most extreme form as vasculitis.

Case Study: Elaine

Elaine had been on every kind of diet, but while the rest of her grew thin and lissom her thighs remained fat and lumpy with cellulite. Exercise made no difference to them either. She was sceptical about the Waterfall Diet, but I explained that she had to use it together with vigorous massage for eight minutes a day. 'Treat your thighs like bread dough' I told her. 'Knead, pummel and squeeze them as much as you can to separate the fluid from the fat. Then the diet will help you get rid of both'. Ten weeks later Elaine's thighs measured 2 inches less in circumference and were getting into proportion with the rest of her body.

Internal Pollution Questionnaire

• Have you noticed an increasing tendency to feel tired most of the time?
• Do you get symptoms such as headaches, drowsiness, coughing or wheezing when exposed to normal amounts of fumes or chemicals such as

dry cleaning or paint fumes, car exhausts, smoke, perfumes, cosmetics or household aerosols and sprays?
• Have you recently started to develop food allergies when you had none before?
• Have you been diagnosed with any of the following illnesses?
  • Arthritis
  • Alzheimer's disease
  • Motor neurone disease
  • Parkinson's disease
  • Kidney disease
  • ME
  • Asthma
  • Psoriasis
• Do you appear to be ageing faster than other people of a similar age?
• Do you normally suffer from a tendency to constipation?
• Do you drink coffee several times a day?
• Do you smoke?
• Are you a medium-to-heavy drinker of alcohol?
• Do you have a lot of amalgam (silver) fillings?
• Do you regularly take medications – even if only aspirin, paracetamol (acetaminophen) or the contraceptive pill?
• Do you consume a lot of processed foods or drinks containing artificial colourings, preservatives and other additives (e.g. dark brown beers, coloured soft drinks or sweets)? If you aren't sure, read the labels: the more E numbers, the more of these undesirable substances are in the food or drink.
• Do you eat less than two portions of fresh fruit or vegetables a day?

If you answered yes to seven or more of the questions above, there is a strong likelihood that your fluid retention may be caused by internal pollution.

Cellulite
At the time of writing, the newspapers are reporting record sales in Australia, of a natural anti-cellulite product called Cellasene.

Based on the herbs ginkgo biloba and clover, and nutrients such as evening primrose oil, fish oil and lecithin, the product was found effective in half the women who tested it in clinical trials there.

Cellulite – a type of body fat found almost exclusively in women, which has a lumpy, dimpled appearance, tends to collect around the thighs and is very hard to shift – can be a big weight problem. The medical profession has divided views about it. Most doctors tell you that it doesn't exist, that it is no different from normal fat and can be lost by dieting and exercising. Some doctors' ears are closed to the women who tell them that this approach simply doesn't work. The doctors who *do* have treatments to offer are plastic surgeons, and they recommend liposuction: physically extracting the offending substance. Cellulite, they confirm, is a type of fat found deep in the skin, its lumpy appearance is due to the uneven distribution of connective tissue below the skin in women – and it does *not* always respond to normal dieting and exercise.

What makes it different?

So far, the only explanation for why cellulite may not burn off like other fat comes from the world of natural medicine. The theory goes like this.

First, we know that only women get cellulite. Second, we know that a combination of a low-calorie diet with a 'cleansing' regime and plenty of vigorous massage can in time get rid of even the most resistant cellulite when ordinary dieting and exercise cannot. Third, we know that a number of toxic substances such as pesticides which we take in through food, air and water dissolve only in fat and not in water. These substances cannot be excreted by your kidneys, and if not properly broken down by your liver will tend to accumulate in your body fat. We also know that the ability of people's livers to break down these toxins and eliminate them from the body can vary 60-fold, so some people will accumulate far more toxins in their body fat than others.

Natural medicine practitioners believe that female hormones

somehow cause a woman's body fat to attract water when it is particularly loaded with toxins. The complex thus formed prevents the fat being broken down when needed for fuel – possibly so that the toxins dissolved in the fat cannot escape into the woman's bloodstream and travel to her reproductive organs, where they might damage her eggs or compromise a possible pregnancy.

How to deal with it the simple way

Only vigorous physical pummelling breaks down these water/fat complexes and releases the water. The fat can then be burned off normally if the body is given a low-calorie diet to encourage its use as fuel. In addition a 'cleansing' regime such as the Waterfall Diet encourages the liver to break down the toxins released from the body fat. This helps prevent them going back into storage all over again.

Because waste from your liver goes to your gall bladder and from there to your intestines, it is also essential to avoid constipation while treating cellulite. Toxins and wastes in your intestinal contents can be reabsorbed through the walls of your intestines into your blood if they have to wait a long time before being evacuated.

Author Liz Hodgkinson has written books describing how it took her only about 12 weeks to rid herself of a severe case of cellulite by following these simple guidelines, the most important part of the treatment being about eight minutes of vigorous massage and pummelling of the problem areas every day. This is certainly worth trying before you opt for liposuction!

If this theory is one day proved, it will mean that cellulite is just another form of fluid retention. If, like many women do, you want to urinate after massaging your problem areas for eight minutes, you have probably released some retained fluid. Try measuring the circumference of your thighs after each massage. You may not get a noticeable difference for a while, but for research purposes I would love to know the results, so please do write to me (see address on p. 210). The fact that cellulite can sometimes be painful if you pinch it also suggests that it may be swollen with retained water.

Of course, even 'dimpled fat' often *does* respond to dieting and exercise. I would like to propose that the more waterlogged it is, the less well it responds. Unfortunately it is impossible to guess how much water cellulite contains just by looking at it, so some research is needed. It would be very interesting to hear from you if massage treatment works for you when nothing else has, especially if at the same time it has made you urinate more than usual.

Anti-cellulite herbs and other products

Natural health products said to aid cellulite reduction are often aromatherapy oil mixtures designed to help stimulate the circulation in the area being massaged. Improved circulation helps to carry the retained fluid away from the area, which in turn helps to improve the transport of nutrients, metabolites (substances created by your body), oxygen and waste products between the fatty tissue and the blood. Anything which helps to bring a warm glow to the area will be useful, so one ingredient of these products may be tiny amounts of pepper oil.

Other products are taken by mouth. These are likely to contain a lot of flavonoids – a type of nutrient found in fruit and vegetables, for instance the white pith of oranges and lemons. As we shall see in Chapter 7, flavonoid deficiency in the diet is one of the commonest causes of fluid retention. The herb ginkgo biloba, found in the product Cellasene, is both rich in flavonoids and has been found in many clinical trials to improve circulation in the capillaries.

Clover flowers are traditionally known as a tonic for the veins and are rich in coumarins, one of the most effective nutrients for reducing some types of fluid retention. There will be more on this in Chapter 7.

Fucus vesiculosis, the seaweed bladderwrack, is added to some anti-cellulite products because of its iodine content. It is not specifically effective against cellulite, but a slight iodine deficiency in your diet can slow your metabolism and make you gain weight, because iodine is vital for the proper functioning of the thyroid gland. People suffering from thyroid deficiency also tend to have myxoedema, a type of fluid retention which occurs in the tissues under the skin and gives it a puffy, waxy appearance. As reported as long ago as 1978 in the medical journal *Clinical Endocrinonology*, thyroid deficiency (*hypothyroidism*) is not always easily diagnosed by a doctor. In this report, the Renal Research Laboratories at the North Staffordshire Medical Institute in England found that out of 11 of their patients with fluid retention, six had antibodies to their thyroid gland, indicating that this gland was damaged. When treated with thyroid hormone supplements, these patients lost their fluid retention. But according to standard medical tests, all the patients had normal thyroid glands. Clearly these tests were not accurate and not sensitive enough. If you have had normal thyroid test results yet have any reason to suspect that you might be hypothyroid, it is worth bullying your doctor to send you for thyroid antibody tests.

So-called 'liver' herbs, such as blue flag or dandelion are sometimes added to anti-cellulite tablets because they help to drain the liver and gall bladder of the processed toxins released from the cellulite. This helps to prevent these wastes from being put back into storage in your body fat, which could perpetuate your cellulite.

Finally one herb, *Centella asiatica* or gotu kola, has undergone some clinical trials on its own for the treatment of cellulite, although the patients were not compared with others using a low-calorie diet alone. In one trial, carried out by Dr A. Dalloz Bourguinon in 1975, a cellulite patient lost $5\frac{1}{2}$ inches (14 cm) from the circumference of her thighs after using gotu kola together with a low-calorie diet for fifty-five days. But the average reduction in thigh circumference for the group of women as a whole was only 1 inch (2.5 cm) during this time, and it is not known whether this might have been achieved with the diet alone.

Gotu kola (which is not related to the kola nut) is found in India, Australia, parts of Africa and the Far East. It is a source of triterpenoid compounds and flavonoids, and has been used as a medicinal herb in India since prehistoric times, and also in

Indonesia, mainly to aid the healing of wounds and to treat leprosy. In China it is favoured as an 'elixir of life' – a herb which promotes long life.

Scientists are interested in the therapeutic benefits of gotu kola, and several medical journals have reported the results of Italian researchers that extracts from this herb act as a skin and blood vessel strengthener, and can treat leaky capillaries, varicose veins and venous insufficiency – a condition where the veins in the legs have difficulty in carrying the blood upwards against the flow of gravity. Perhaps this type of circulatory problem contributes to the development of the more severe forms of cellulite.

Internal Pollution and Vasculitis

You may have wondered why the questionnaire on pp. 61–2 asks whether you are sensitive to chemicals such as car exhausts, dry cleaning fumes, cigarette smoke or perfume. Chemical sensitivity is usually a good indicator that the liver is overloaded with internal pollution and that you are at risk of developing fluid retention as a result.

Environmental medicine

Doctors who specialize in environmental medicine – the investigation of sensitivity to foods and to chemicals in our environment as a possible explanation for illnesses in patients who do not get well in the normal way – treat it by reducing the patient's usually high levels of internal pollution. First they carry out liver function tests to see which chemicals it is processing too sluggishly. The reason for the sluggishness is usually a lack of enzymes (substances produced by the body, assisted by specific nutrients, which help it convert one chemical into another). In turn, the enzymes are thought to be deficient because that person's body needs larger than usual amounts of those nutrients.

Once the deficient enzymes have been identified, extra amounts of the appropriate nutrients are given together with a low-allergen diet and strict environmental control – preventing any more unwanted chemicals from entering the patient's body for a while. This type of approach can result in a return to health in seemingly hopeless cases of vasculitis as well as asthma, severe chronic fatigue, Gulf War syndrome and autoimmune diseases such as rheumatoid arthritis. (Autoimmune diseases are usually serious illnesses in which the cells of the immune system begin attacking the body's own organs and tissues because they begin to appear abnormal.)

Success with treating vasculitis

One of the greatest advocates and practitioners of environmental medicine today, Dr William Rea from Dallas, carried out a very interesting research study in 1976 on ten vasculitis sufferers. Vasculitis means inflammation of the blood vessels, and one of its symptoms is recurrent fluid retention. Others are bruising and red marks around the affected vessels.

Dr Rea recorded all these patients' symptoms, looking for signs of allergy and chemical sensitivity. Apart from their symptoms of vasculitis all the patients also suffered from recurrent nasal stuffiness and susceptibility to cold. Most had muscle pains, sinusitis and regular headaches. Half had recurrent overwhelming fatigue and sore throats. Some also suffered from asthma, depression and cystitis. Most had had these illnesses for about twenty years, and had seen at least ten doctors before consulting Dr Rea.

Dr Rea reasoned that since so many of these problems can be symptoms of allergic illness or chemical sensitivity, perhaps the vasculitis was too. He put the patients into a controlled environment where they could be kept away from all modern chemicals, and stopped their food and medications for a few days.

It took only four or five days for all the patients' symptoms to clear. Then they were 'challenged' with normal, chemically grown foods, tap water and the usual variety of everyday chemicals to which most of us are exposed: formaldehyde gas from soft furnishings, cigarette smoke, natural gas, chlorine and so on. The vasculitis and fluid retention reappeared in every case when small amounts of these chemicals were inhaled.

Although this study was reported in the medical journal *Annals of Allergy*, it and others like it have, amazingly enough, been ignored by the medical profession, despite the dangers and comparative ineffectiveness of the drug-based treatments which are still the norm. It is most unlikely that any doctor you might consult would use this approach if you should need it. If you wish to find a doctor like Dr Rea or Dr Monro, who is mentioned on page 70, see Useful Addresses on p. 202.

A possible explanation

But how could inhaling or consuming small amounts of chemicals cause inflammation of the blood vessels, bruising, swelling and fluid retention? Vasculitis is normally caused by the immune system reacting to a bacterial infection, or by an irritating drug. At the time of this research Dr Rea did not know the answer, but he knew that the signs of bruising meant that tiny blood capillaries were being ruptured.

Dr John Gerrard, Professor of Pediatrics at the University of Saskatchewan in Canada, writes in his book *Food Allergy: New Perspectives*, that he may have an explanation. The walls of blood vessels have an affinity 15 times greater than the rest of the body for a very common type of toxic chemical known as phenol. (Plastic, among other things, is made from phenols.) This in itself only means that phenols will tend to collect in blood vessel walls. But if it does, will the cells of the vessel walls still be recognizable to the immune system? If they are not, the immune system may mount an attack against them. This type of immune attack against the body's own cells happens very frequently. We also know that many chemical substances such as formaldehyde, PVC and acetone have been shown to trigger the kinin system – a mechanism of the immune system which can cause pain and inflammation in blood vessels.

As we shall see later, vasculitis can also occur from a type of tissue damage called crosslinking, when the wrong amino acids join up with each other. Crosslinking occurs when toxic chemicals begin to build up in the body, either because there are too many for the liver to deal with or because the liver has become sluggish in dealing with them. Too much crosslinking in the body is destructive to a lot of its important functions.

Internal Pollution and Your Liver

To help prevent fluid retention caused by internal pollution, it is important to know a little about your liver, whose task it is to keep down your pollution levels. Some livers are better at this job than others. We have already mentioned that the ability of different people's livers to detoxify pesticides and other toxic substances taken in through our food, air and water, can vary as much as 60-fold. This means that one person who smokes 60 cigarettes a day and whose liver is very efficient at detoxifying the cancer-causing substances in cigarette smoke, for example, may be no more likely to get cancer than another who smokes only one cigarette a day, or one who is even a passive smoker, but has a particularly inefficient liver.

The problem is that we have no way of knowing how efficient our liver is before we start smoking or before we realize that environmental toxins are affecting our health. We may have no idea that our liver is letting us down until we notice signs that our body is in a state of toxic overload – that is to say, suffering from 'internal pollution'. Have another look at the questionnaire on pp. 61–2 to remind yourself of some of these signs and the ways you yourself may be placing an extra burden on your liver, and perhaps encouraging cellulite or vasculitis.

Dr Jean Monro of the Breakspear Hospital in the UK, who specializes in the treatment of people with illnesses caused by chemical sensitivity, has found that the livers of up to 58 per cent of her patients have difficulty in processing even mildly toxic substances like caffeine. As we shall see later, these livers are not diseased but overworked and undernourished. Giving them more of the nutrients they need can in time help them to function better and cope with a normal workload.

If you suffer from cellulite, vasculitis or any related fluid retention caused by internal pollution, your liver will need all the help you can give it. Do remember that your liver is completely dependent on you to look after it. It has no-one else in the world but you.

How the Liver Works

Many of the waste products found in your blood, as well as toxins ingested in your food, air and water, or as drugs and medicines, cannot be directly excreted by your kidneys. This is either because your kidneys keep reabsorbing them or because they do not dissolve in water. Your liver's job is to change them until they do dissolve in water and so can be excreted in your urine or (via your gall bladder) through your bowels. This is usually known as 'detoxification', but more correctly as biotransformation – the transforming of one substance into another, more excretable one.

Liver detox Phase I

There are two main phases of liver biotransformation. In Phase I unwanted chemicals are made to undergo chemical reactions such as oxidation (combining them with oxygen).

Eventually, step by step, liver enzymes turn the chemicals into intermediates, and then into acids. Since these acids are water-soluble, they can be extracted from your blood by your kidneys and excreted from your body.

It does not follow that, as your liver acts on the unwanted chemicals, they become less and less toxic. In fact, the intermediate chemicals created during Phase I can sometimes be far more toxic than the original ones. Cigarette smoke is an example. Your body will be able to neutralize some of these toxins with antioxidants – vitamins C and E, flavonoids and beta carotene, or with enzymes which do a similar job. The bigger your liver's workload, the more toxic intermediate products will be made, and the more antioxidants will be used up. For instance, it may surprise you to know that smokers use vitamin C twice as fast as other people. Because their liver is coping with so much extra toxicity, they need to consume twice as much vitamin C as non-smokers just to maintain the same amount of this important protective nutrient in their blood.

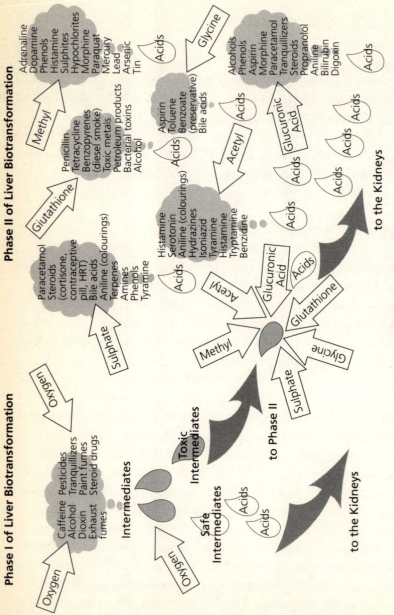

Some examples of the above-mentioned harmful intermediate toxins include:

- free radicals
- aldehydes
- epoxides
- chloral hydrate (identical to the knock-out drops known as the 'Mickey Finn') and even
- Valium-like compounds.

Some of the well-known chemicals which have to go through Phase I biotransformation by your liver include:

- caffeine
- alcohol
- dioxin (a pollutant)
- exhaust fumes
- organophosphorous pesticides
- paint fumes
- steroid hormones
- drugs including paracetamol (acetaminophen), diazepam tranquillizers and sleeping pills, the contraceptive pill and cortisone.

The more of these you ingest, the more Phase I enzymes your liver must produce, and the more antioxidants you will need.

Liver overload
But what happens if for some reason there aren't enough enzymes and antioxidants to go round?

Basically, the Phase I process will stop somewhere along the line. The intermediate chemicals that we mentioned earlier: free radicals, aldehydes, epoxides, chloral hydrate and Valium-like compounds will begin to build up. Can you guess how these substances will make you feel as their levels rise? People have reported feeling 'hung-over' all the time, or drowsy, or suffering from depression and irritability, fluid retention, problems with concentrating, or fatigue. Often people feel all right for most of the time, but exposure to slightly larger amounts of chemicals can tip the balance again, bringing back the symptoms.

This is the condition described earlier – chemical sensitivity. If you have it, as time goes by more and more chemicals could begin to affect you – eventually even the natural chemicals occurring in food and drink, such as natural insecticides in plants, and ammonia from consuming protein. If you come to associate your symptoms with eating particular foods, you may believe that you have a food intolerance (as described in Chapter 2), but in fact the symptoms are a warning sign that your liver is overloaded.

The difference between a food intolerance and a sensitivity to the natural chemicals in food is that in most cases of food intolerance only one or two foods will make you feel ill. With a chemical sensitivity, however, you feel ill most of the time, because it is virtually impossible to avoid all the common chemicals with which we are surrounded.

The symptoms you experience depend on which type of intermediate chemical is building up in your system. Free radicals cause cells to die by rupturing their delicate protective outer membranes. Epoxides damage brain cells and increase the risk of cancer. Aldehydes (which are also found in cheap wine) cause headaches and, in the most severe cases, protein crosslinking and inflammation of the blood vessels or even epilepsy. Chloral hydrate and Valium-like compounds affect your concentration and can make you feel tired or drowsy.

Secondary reactions (usually involving histamine and inflammation), as the immune system is activated in the parts of the body harbouring these chemicals, vary from person to person. Depending on where they become concentrated, they can cause anything from migraine to arthritis, asthma, vasculitis, fluid retention and skin reactions with rashes and swellings.

If this pattern of very poor health sounds like you, your liver may be in need of a helping hand.

Liver detox Phase II

Phase II of the liver's detoxification work involves combining unwanted chemicals with one of five main types of substances:

- sulphate
- acetyl groups
- methyl groups
- glucuronic acid
- amino acids

The goal is still the same: to make the chemicals dissolve in water so that they can be excreted by the kidneys. Different chemicals are processed in different ways. So while caffeine is fully broken down by Phase I, paracetamol has to be combined with sulphate, and aspirin with glycine in Phase II.

The disturbances caused to the body's metabolism by excessive internal pollution may be an explanation for the modern plague of chronic illnesses. Work carried out in recent years in England at Birmingham University by Dr Guy Steventon and Dr Rosemary Waring has shown that the livers of many people with M.E. (chronic fatigue syndrome), parkinsonism, motor neurone disease (also known as ALS) and Alzheimer's disease are more sluggish than those of healthy people in dealing with internal pollution. Similar work has been carried out at the University of Cincinnati in relation to bladder cancer. All this research has been published in several medical journals, including *Nature* and the *Lancet*, but little attention is being paid to it in the medical world because of its lack of commercial potential. If research could be done to measure the liver function of several thousand healthy people and observe which of these develop the above-mentioned diseases over the next 20 years, this subject would be more difficult to ignore, but who is going to fund it?

Giving Your Liver a Helping Hand

If all this sounds rather daunting, don't worry! It is only intended to give you insights into the causes of any ill health and fluid retention which you already know that you suffer from, and to encourage you to work towards a healthier lifestyle. The Waterfall Diet is a lifestyle change *par excellence* which can not only help your fluid retention but increase your chances of living an active, happy old age rather than the average unhealthy old age suffered by so many. And it really is never too late to start. If your liver is a little sluggish, the Waterfall Diet can help it. Some care and attention and extra nutrients can make all the difference.

The right foods
Foods which are good for the other organs of the body are good for the liver too. We can also use diet to help our liver by eating foods which:

- keep to a minimum the amount of unwanted chemicals which our liver has to deal with
- reduce the absorption of unwanted chemicals from the intestines into the bloodstream
- nourish the biotransformation enzymes
- provide abundant raw materials for unwanted chemicals to combine with in Phase II
- are rich in antioxidants which help to reduce the toxicity of the intermediate chemicals which the liver forms
- help the liver to produce its own antioxidant enzymes
- help to drain wastes from the liver by stimulating the gall bladder to empty.

The Waterfall Diet has been designed with this in mind, and the appropriate foods are listed in the table on p. 77.

Constipation and its implications
Foods high in dietary fibre are especially important for preventing one of the causes of internal pollution – constipation. Generally speaking, fibre is the indigestible part of our food, such as bran, cellulose and tough vegetable fibres and skins. Gum-like substances found in beans and seeds, and pectin which is found

Foods and Nutrients Which Assist The Liver

Food/Nutrient	Biotransformation Used In	Cellular Repair and Protection	Liver and Gall Bladder Drainage
Brassicas (broccoli, cauliflower, brussels sprouts, cabbage)	Phase I	Milk thistle herb (or its extract silymarin)	Beetroot juice
N-acetyl cysteine (NAC)[1]	Phase I. Also needed to make glutathione	Turmeric (yellow Indian spice)	Radish juice
Antioxidants (vitamins C & E, beta carotene)	Neutralizing dangerous free radicals produced in Phase I		Watercress
Selenium[2]	Forming the antioxidant enzyme glutathione peroxidase		Dandelion coffee
Manganese[2]	Forming the antioxidant enzyme superoxide dismutase (SOD)		Golden seal (herb)
Sulphate[2]	Combining toxins with sulphur in Phase II		Milk thistle herb (or its extract silymarin)
Molybdenum[2]	Sulphoxidation (sulphate production)		
Pantothenic acid (vitamin B5)	Combining toxins with acetyl[3] in Phase I.		
Methionine[1]	Combining toxins with methyl[3] in Phase I.		

77

Magnesium[2]	Ditto
Protein	Combining toxins with protein in Phase I.
Gelatine (consists of one third glycine[1])	Combining toxins with glycine in Phase I.
Taurine[1]	Combining toxins with taurine in Phase I.
Reduced glutathione[1]	Combining toxins with glutathione in Phase I.

[1] An amino acid
[2] A mineral
[3] Units of carbon used in body processes

in fruit, are also classified as dietary fibre. Fibre can absorb several times its weight in water and so it softens the stools and adds bulk. Your large intestine, or colon, needs this softness and bulk in order to move its contents towards the rectum, from which they can be evacuated.

Besides fibre and water, your stools contain waste products excreted by your liver into your gall bladder (which empties into your intestines), toxins produced by the many bacteria which reside in your intestine, and millions of dead bacteria. As this mixture of substances, known as faeces, enters your colon it is quite liquid. One of the colon's jobs is to extract water from the faeces and to return it to the bloodstream, together with substances dissolved in it. Your body is only interested in useful dissolved substances such as vitamins and mineral salts. Unfortunately harmful wastes and bacterial toxins can also be absorbed back into your blood along with the water. The longer it takes for your faeces to be expelled in a bowel motion, the more unwanted substances can be reabsorbed in this way. This adds to your liver's workload just like any other source of internal pollution.

Bran may help you to have bowel motions, but sometimes only because it irritates your bowels slightly so that they want to get rid of it as soon as possible. Eating a wide variety of wholegrains, beans and fresh fruit and vegetables, as in the Waterfall Diet, is the best way to get all the different types of dietary fibre that your body needs. It will also ensure that you benefit from the huge variety of nutrients found in these foods. By nutrients I don't just mean vitamins, minerals, starches and proteins, but essential polyunsaturated oils, flavonoids, carotenes and sterols now known to play important roles in maintaining good health and preventing diseases.

Of the vegetables, broccoli, cauliflower and cabbage help the liver with its biotransformation work, while beetroot, radishes and watercress help to drain your liver by stimulating your gall bladder – a tiny storage organ under your liver into which your liver empties its waste products – to empty itself into your intestines. Beetroot juice has been recommended by naturopaths for a hundred years for this beneficial effect.

Why not add the bright yellow culinary herb known as turmeric, often found in Indian curries, to your cooking for its protective effect on your liver cells? The medicinal herb milk thistle also protects liver cells from damage and helps to regenerate the liver if any previous damage has occurred. Many research studies on milk thistle and its extract silymarin have now been carried out with excellent results.

Will Fasting Help Your Liver?

Although some books on naturopathy still recommend fasting as a technique to 'cleanse' the liver, we now know more about the functioning of the liver. While fasting may be useful to rest the digestive system when it is overstressed, it makes you quickly burn off body fat which contains stored toxins. The faster your body fat is burned off, the faster these toxins are released into your blood. Once these toxins are released they have to be processed by your liver, but the liver cannot do this without a supply of protein. So if you have any symptoms of chemical sensitivity your protein intake *must* be kept up if your overall calorie intake drops – otherwise your symptoms could worsen as the build-up of intermediate toxic chemicals increases.

Are Dietary Supplements Worth Taking?

Environmental medicine experts make great use of dietary supplements to help with the liver's biotransformation processes. The nutrients most needed can be determined with special liver function tests that use a 'marker' substance like caffeine or aspirin to measure how well each part (or pathway) of the biotransformation process takes place in your body.

You consume a precise quantity of the marker substance. When broken down by a normal liver it should result within a few hours in the appearance of a particular end product (metabolite) in your urine. A sample of your urine is collected at a specific time, and the amounts of this metabolite are measured. If they are found to be too low, the particular process in your liver which is responsible for breaking down this type of unwanted chemical is faulty.

Sometimes only one of these processes is faulty, sometimes all. Each process is dependent on a range of nutrients and can often be improved when their intake is increased. Pollution of all types really does increase our need for many vitamins, minerals, amino acids and other nutrients. It may be possible to get the necessary improvement in liver function just by eating a better diet. On the other hand some people with this problem already eat an excellent diet but are not absorbing their nutrients very well. Sometimes the body even has problems in forming the more complex nutrients which it must make itself, such as taurine, glutathione, GLA and EPA. Using supplements as an added precaution ensures that nothing is left to chance, and is very unlikely to cause harm.

Sources of Chemicals in Your Environment

There are sixty thousand chemicals in current commercial production. Three thousand of these are used as food additives, and eight hundred are found in drinking water. All can contribute to your internal pollution. Pollutants can be absorbed from:

- traffic fumes, especially carcinogenic particles in diesel smoke and lead from petrol
- factory and power station discharges into air, rivers and seas
- fish caught in polluted waters, especially in coastal areas
- food contaminated with pesticides
- industrial fall-out (particles which were originally in fumes or smoke and have subsequently settled on crops which feed us and the animals we subsequently eat)
- invisible clouds of pesticide which can be blown halfway across the world for us to breathe in. Pesticide is sprayed on pavements and parks, used in gardens, contained in wood preservatives, used on footpaths, road margins and in buildings. It is washed into the water table which provides our drinking water

We can also bring pollution into our own homes by the products and services we use:

- artificial air fresheners
- artificial food additives
- cosmetic aerosols and sprays, e.g. deodorant, hairspray, perfume
- dry cleaning fumes
- dust
- fly spray and other insecticides
- formaldehyde gas released by new carpets and furnishings (see the main text for some of the harmful effects of this and other types of aldehydes)
- fumes from garages built underneath bedrooms or adjacent to living quarters
- fumes from gas cookers and central heating
- garden sprays
- household sprays
- mould from damp surroundings
- re-used cooking oil (increases levels of harmful peroxides in food)

- soap powders and detergents made from strong chemicals
- strong-smelling fabric conditioners
- strong-smelling polishes, toilet cleaners and carpet cleaners
- tobacco smoke
- unnecessary medications or recreational drugs
- wood preservative

The human body can also become polluted with chemicals produced by too many of the wrong kinds of resident bacteria in the intestines. The fatigue and foggy thinking suffered by people with an overgrowth of *Candida albicans*, for example, may be due to the harmful aldehydes produced by this yeast.

CHAPTER

Your Personal Plumbing System: Looking after Your Blood and Lymph Vessels

There are an estimated 25,000 miles of blood vessels in your body

This chapter explains the normal processes of fluid exchange between your blood vessels and the cells of your muscles, organs and other tissues, and what actually happens at this level when things go wrong. It also looks at another important cause of fluid retention: congestion of your lymphatic system, whose job it is to collect excess fluid and return it to your blood.

Case Study: John

John was a couch potato. Unemployed, he sat around at home all day or lay in bed, watching TV and reading the newspaper. In the evenings he would visit friends, or they would come to see him, and enjoy a few cans of lager sitting around watching TV. Occasionally John went to the pub. He did not play any sports or take any other form of exercise.

Needless to say, John was getting more and more overweight. But when he tried a low-calorie diet for a while, it didn't seem to make much difference. Then John got a job packing shelves in a supermarket, and within days the weight was falling off him. His previous lack of activity had slowed down his lymphatic system so much that fluid was not properly draining out of his tissue spaces but was collecting and adding to his weight problem. Once he got a job, the extra activity activated John's lymphatic system and the fluid was able to drain away.

Answer the following questionnaire to see whether your fluid retention is due to problems with your blood capillaries or lymphatic vessels:

Capillary and Lymphatic Questionnaire

- Do you eat fresh fruit or vegetables less than once a day?
- If you are a woman, do you suffer from heavy periods?
- Do you bruise easily?
- Do you suffer from broken capillaries or thread veins?
- Do you avoid physical exercise?
- Do you sit still for several hours every day, for instance watching TV?
- Are you bed- or wheelchair-bound?

If you answered yes to two or more of the first four questions, there is a strong possibility that your fluid retention is caused by leaky blood vessels. If you answered yes to any of the last three questions, your fluid retention may be caused or aggravated by lymphatic congestion.

The 'Pipework' of Your Body (1): The Circulation of the Blood

Imagine that the fluid system in your body is similar to the one in your home – with mains pipes taking the fluid to smaller pipes, which carry the fluid to outlets; and a drainage network to carry away the waste water. In your body the mains pipes are known as arteries; they are large and carry oxygen-rich arterial blood consisting of:

- red and white blood cells, platelet cells
- plasma, a clear, watery fluid which contains dissolved nutrients and other substances.

Arterial blood is a very bright red because it has recently come from your lungs, where oxygen attaches to its red cells, changing their colour. Arterial blood has also recently come from your heart, which exerts a tremendous pumping pressure (so if one of your arteries is severed, blood comes out with great force). This pressure is necessary to get the blood, and the oxygen and nutrients it contains, to all parts of your body.

Arteries, capillaries, tissues and cells

Arteries branch off into smaller and smaller versions of themselves. Small arteries are known as arterioles. The tiniest branches of all – hardly visible to the naked eye – are called capillaries, and there are an estimated 25,000 miles of them in your body. Your capillaries take blood to your tissues – the 'fabric' of your body, which consists of many kinds of cells. Examples are heart tissue, liver tissue, skin tissue and muscle tissue. A cell is the smallest unit of living matter.

How fluid moves via the capillaries

Your capillaries do not have 'taps' to let fluid out of them, but they do have a controlled filter system built into their walls. The filter allows fluid from your blood to escape from the capillaries into your tissue spaces – the gaps between your cells. As your cells become bathed in this fluid, they take up the oxygen and nutrients dissolved in it and in return discharge their own waste products into it. Once the fluid enters your tissue spaces it is called tissue fluid or extracellular fluid. The tissue spaces have a very large capacity for holding fluid, and if you suffer from fluid retention this is the place where excess fluid builds up and collects.

As waste products from your cells collect in your tissue fluid, the filter in your capillary walls allows the fluid to re-enter your capillary system so that it can be taken to your liver and kidneys for the wastes to be processed and eliminated. The capillaries which will accept this waste-filled fluid are known as the venous capillaries; they eventually link up to another set of large blood vessels, your veins, which take blood back to your heart. Any excess fluid not removed from tissue spaces by your venous

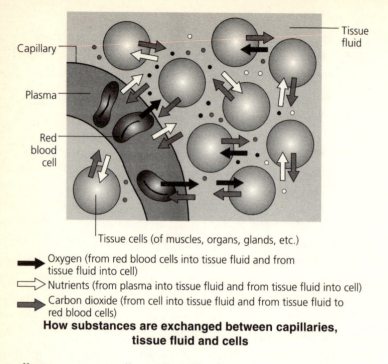

Tissue fluid

Capillary

Plasma

Red blood cell

Tissue cells (of muscles, organs, glands, etc.)

→ Oxygen (from red blood cells into tissue fluid and from tissue fluid into cell)

⇒ Nutrients (from plasma into tissue fluid and from tissue fluid into cell)

→ Carbon dioxide (from cell into tissue fluid and from tissue fluid to red blood cells)

How substances are exchanged between capillaries, tissue fluid and cells

capillaries is normally collected up and removed by your lymphatic system – a different network, which, as we shall see on p. 91, plays a very important part in preventing fluid retention.

While the blood in arteries and arterial capillaries is bright red and full of oxygen and nutrients, the blood in your veins and venous capillaries is dark and full of waste products and carbon dioxide. The two blood systems are not separate; arterial capillaries eventually become venous capillaries, which then grow larger to become veins. Eventually the veins reach your heart, which pumps the blood to your lungs and then, further supplies of oxygen into your arteries again.

What Decides How Much Fluid Enters Your Tissue Spaces?

Your body tries to maintain a balance between the contents of your blood plasma and the fluid in your tissue spaces. For example, if your tissue fluid contains a lot of glucose, your plasma will hold on to its glucose until more of the glucose in your tissue fluid has passed into your cells. On the other hand, if glucose levels in your tissue fluid are low, then glucose-rich plasma arriving after a meal will quickly lose its glucose to the tissue fluid until glucose levels are evenly balanced in both fluids.

This works in the other direction, too. Only if levels of the cells' waste product carbon dioxide are higher in the tissue fluid than in the blood plasma will carbon dioxide be able to pass into the capillaries. The same applies to water. Dilute fluid will tend to flow in the direction of concentrated fluid in order to even things up, and vice versa. So at times when your tissue fluid is more concentrated than your blood, more fluid will tend to flow out of your capillaries into your tissue spaces.

The volume of fluid in your tissue spaces should be three to four times greater than the volume of your plasma. (In fact, in a 14 stone (200 lb) man, half his body weight consists of his cells while the other half consists of the material in his tissue spaces.) This balance between plasma and tissue fluid is maintained by three principal mechanisms:

- the difference in fluid pressure on either side of your capillary walls
- the permeability ('leakiness') of your capillary walls
- the difference between the protein concentrations in your plasma and those in your tissue fluid.

So excess fluid in your tissue spaces should normally be drawn into your venous capillaries, because the blood pressure in them is low and your plasma normally contains high levels of proteins, which have a strong water-pulling force. In spite of this, in the course of a day your capillary arteries transfer more than 5 pints more fluid to the tissue spaces than the capillary veins can re-absorb. Because this extra tissue fluid cannot filter back into your bloodstream by itself, it is collected and returned to the bloodstream by your lymphatic system.

We saw in Chapter 3, that an exceptionally low-protein diet can cause fluid retention. This is because it results in low protein levels in your plasma, reducing the plasma's water-pulling force and leaving fluid to accumulate in your tissue spaces.

Fluid retention can occur when any of the three balancing mechanisms listed above are disturbed. Let's take a look at how they can go wrong.

Fluid Pressure Problems

Lots of things can affect your fluid balance by interfering with the pressure on either side of your capillary walls. For example, hormones such as adrenaline, acetylcholine and angiotensin can make your blood pressure go up or down by dilating or constricting your arterioles. This may be important in stress situations, for instance, when your muscles need a greater blood supply than normal. Adrenaline sends your blood pressure up by constricting the blood vessels at the outer edges of your body and enabling more blood to be concentrated around your muscles, helping you to run away from, or fight, your source of stress.

In a healthy body most pressure changes are only temporary, and have no long-term effect on your tissue fluid. On the other hand, a blockage or congestion of your veins, or a failure of your heart to pump adequately, can cause long-term pressure changes which permanently reduce your capillaries' ability to absorb water back from your tissue fluid. These situations can cause serious fluid retention and weight gain.

Congestive heart failure

This illness, which results in severe swelling, has a 'double whammy' effect on fluid retention. Poor pumping action by the heart reduces the flow of blood through the kidneys. This fools the body into thinking that its total fluid levels are low rather than high, so it steps up production of the salt-retention hormone aldosterone. When salt (sodium) is retained, the kidneys hold on to water instead of excreting it. Urination diminishes and tissue fluid levels rise, especially in the feet and ankles – the parts of your body where the fluid pressure is greatest due to the effects of gravity. Your feet and ankles can become so swollen that you need to wear support stockings and may have to buy shoes several sizes larger than usual.

If you have been diagnosed with this condition, see a nutritionist for special advice on natural remedies which can help you in addition to the Waterfall Diet.

Capillary Wall Permeability

The permeability of a capillary wall is its ability to let fluid, protein and other substances through it. In a healthy person this permeability is strictly controlled. But if your capillary walls somehow become too 'leaky', excess protein can escape into your tissue fluid. Since protein attracts fluid, more fluid will flow from your capillaries into your tissue spaces, resulting in fluid retention. As fluid leaves your blood, your body will try to normalize your blood volume by making more of the sodium-retaining hormone aldosterone. Your kidneys will then excrete less fluid, thus worsening the fluid retention. Capillary health and strength is therefore very important indeed to prevent fluid retention.

What makes capillary walls too leaky?

Factors which can make your capillary walls more leaky include:

- shock
- infections
- damage to your capillaries by physical injury (e.g. bruising, friction or radiation)
- damage to your capillaries by nutritional deficiencies which make your blood vessels more fragile
- imbalances in the production of hormone-like substances known as prostaglandins (see p. 113).

An example of fluid leakage from damaged capillaries is the blister effect. Friction from a badly-fitting shoe, for instance, or heat from a burn, damages the capillaries under your skin. These leak fluid under the surface layer of your skin, forming a blister.

Histamine, a chemical released when allergic reactions occur, can have a similar effect to an injury on your capillary walls. It causes the junctions between the cells comprising your capillary walls to widen temporarily, allowing fluid to leak out into your tissue spaces.

Signs of leaky capillaries include a tendency:

- to bruise too easily
- to suffer extensively from thread (spider) veins or little red blood marks under the skin
- in women, to suffer from heavy periods.

How to keep capillaries in good condition

It is vital to give your capillary walls enough of the nutrients they need to keep them strong and healthy. These nutrients, vitamin C and flavonoids (see p. 116) are found in fruit and vegetables. The white 'pithy' part of oranges is especially helpful, as it is very rich in flavonoids. Although there are, of course, other causes of heavy periods, this problem is sometimes associated with a very low intake of fresh fruits and vegetables and in this case it can be cleared up by consuming more of them. As so often happens with foods, the most nutritious parts are the parts we tend to throw away! If you do not eat fresh fruit and vegetables every day, you could be at risk of fluid retention.

In one scientific study carried out in France, a treatment based on supplementation with flavonoids was successfully used to treat fifteen cases of fluid retention caused by excessively leaky capillaries.

But treating damaged capillaries with flavonoids is not a new notion. The importance of these nutrients in capillary health has been known for 50 years. Several scientific studies in the 1950s found that capillary damage caused by treatment with radiation could be much reduced by supplementing the diet with vitamin C and/or flavonoids. It is odd that radiotherapy patients do not seem to be told this by their doctor or radiotherapist.

Protein Concentration Imbalances

For correct fluid balance, the differences between the protein concentration in the blood plasma in your capillaries, and that in your tissue fluid, must be carefully maintained. Over-permeable capillary walls can leak protein into your tissue fluid. As the protein levels build up in your tissue spaces, they attract water from your bloodstream which cannot be returned unless the protein levels are reduced.

As we saw above and in Chapter 6, there are all sorts of reasons why capillary walls can become leaky. But provided the amount of extra protein in the tissue fluid is not too great, all is not necessarily lost. Your lymphatic system can return some protein from the tissue fluid to your bloodstream – a routine part of its work. Although most healthy capillaries only have a slight permeability to protein, there is still a small, steady movement of protein from your blood into your tissue fluid. It is only when your lymphatics fail to remove it – by carrying away the tissue fluid containing it – that the concentration of protein in your tissue fluid will rise.

So congestion of your lymphatic vessels, resulting in failure to do this important job, is another potential cause of fluid retention. This type of fluid retention is known as lymphoedema.

The 'Pipework' of Your Body (2): The Lymphatic System

Lymph vessels are present in almost every organ of the body, and are extremely important in preventing fluid retention. As we have seen, they help to drain away any excess tissue fluid which the capillaries cannot absorb. These vessels have very thin walls and large pores: they easily absorb tissue fluid since they are permeable to all its constituents, including protein.

Once your tissue fluid enters your lymphatic system it is known as lymph and is channelled through your lymph vessels, which converge to form ever-larger vessels. The two largest drain into veins in your neck, thus returning the fluid to your bloodstream. A blockage of your lymphatic system can cause severe fluid retention by preventing the return of excess tissue fluid to your blood.

Exercise is important for lymph vessels

Unlike your blood circulation, lymph has no heart to pump it around. Lymph flow depends on the massaging effect produced by using the muscles through which your lymph vessels flow, and there are valves to make the lymph flow only in one direction – towards the points at which the lymph vessels enter your blood system. Regular exercise is therefore one of the few things which will stimulate lymphatic flow. And the automatic rhythmic contractions of the muscle tissue that surrounds your larger lymphatic vessels exert a pump-like action which has a stimulating effect.

One reason why long-distance flights can cause fluid retention is the fact that passengers have to sit in cramped conditions, virtually immobile, for hours on end. Complete bed-rest can cause devastating fluid retention, which hospital staff usually try to prevent by making patients get up regularly even after major surgery. And the modern couch potato lifestyle is responsible for a type of fluid retention known as television oedema. All movement helps to prevent the problem. Even if just your foot is moved, the lymphatic vessels in your leg can fill up much more effectively than if your foot is completely still.

Massage is valuable too

If exercise is impossible, the next most effective way to stimulate your lymphatic circulation is with massage. This does not have to be vigorous. Your lymph vessels are delicate and can be damaged if you massage too vigorously. See the diagram on p. 100 for the correct massage points and directions. One reason why we automatically massage ourselves when we have received a bump or bruise is because we unconsciously know that this is a good way to stimulate the lymphatic system around the injured part.

Injuries can sometimes develop quite serious fluid retention, which makes them even more painful. When I was involved in a minor car accident I severely wrenched one of my fingers and suffered pain and swelling around one of the joints for nearly a year afterwards. Regular massage helped to drain away the fluid which was causing the problem. The fact that it took so long for the swelling to go down is not unusual, according to lymphologists – doctors who specialize in disorders of the lymphatic system. As described on p. 94, fluid retention can sometimes actually be a *cause* of inflammation.

Fluid retention under the eyes, producing baggy lower eyelids, occurs when tissues are excessively compliant; that is to say, as they absorb more fluid, not enough pressure builds up in them to drive the excess into the lymphatic system. So if you suffer from this problem the delicate tissues under your eyes need a little assistance from you. All tissues can be weakened by a lack of vitamin C or by failure to consume enough flavonoids from fruit and vegetables, so the Waterfall Diet includes plenty of these nutrients. Daily gentle massage, not just around your eyes but of your face, neck and armpits too, will help your lymphatic system to drain the under-eye area. Do ensure as well that you get enough exercise, especially of your upper body – for instance, daily arm swinging and head-rolling exercises.

Your lymph is filtered by lymph nodes positioned in your neck, armpits, groin, tummy and other places. If these nodes are removed by surgery, or if they become inflamed or hardened (fibrosed), your flow of lymph can become blocked. If this occurs in an arm or leg, that limb could become swollen while the rest of your body remains normal.

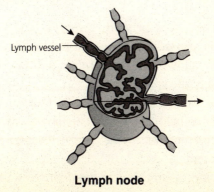

Lymph vessel

Lymph node

Inflammation and Your Lymphatic System

While fluid retention is often the result of inflammation, another kind, known as high-protein type fluid retention, probably also causes it. It occurs when blood capillaries leak so much protein into the tissue spaces that the lymphatic system cannot carry enough of it away. Since protein attracts water, water is then drawn into the tissue spaces.

Accumulations of protein from the blood plasma in the tissues are known to have an irritating, inflammatory effect on the surrounding tissues, causing redness and swelling. Long-term inflammation eventually damages these tissues. High-protein type fluid retention probably has a similar effect, according to the experts.

This area of research has been written about extensively by Dr John Casley-Smith, Past President of the International Society for Lymphology, working at the University of Adelaide in Australia. In his book *High Protein Oedemas And The Benzo-pyrones*, he explains that the main causes of high-protein type fluid retention are:

- Injury to the blood vessels: either a physical injury such as a blow, sprain or excessive friction, or chemical damage of the type described in Chapter 6. For instance a single exposure to an irritant like the weed-killer Paraquat has been known to cause long-term high-protein type fluid retention. If the irritant is inhaled as fumes, the fluid retention might occur in the lungs.
- Widening of the gaps between the cells which comprise the capillary walls, caused by the release of histamine from allergic reactions. This allows fluid and protein to leak out of the capillaries into the tissue spaces.
- Weakening of the blood vessel walls by nutritional deficiencies, particularly vitamins B and C and the flavonoids.
- Injuries or obstructions to the fluid-collecting section of the lymphatic system.
- Lack of exercise to stimulate the lymphatic system.

So what might be described as a case of arthritis, for example, with redness and swelling around a joint, and the destruction of the surrounding cartilage, could have started off as a case of high-protein type fluid retention caused by stress to weakened blood vessels around the joint. If the lymphatic system was not then able to carry away the excess protein, this protein could eventually cause long-term inflammation with resulting damage to the joint tissue. Chilblains which take a long time to heal and eventually cause slight deformities like enlarged finger joints are another example. Chilblains are probably caused by a combination of nutritional deficiencies which make blood capillaries too fragile and then easily injured when cold fingers or toes are placed too close to a fire or radiator.

What Damage Does Long-term Inflammation Cause?

Fibrosis
First, it can result in a hardening of the tissues known as fibrosis, which:

- prevents fluid getting to the lymphatic system
- makes it harder for fluid to travel through the lymphatic system once there
- makes it difficult for white blood cells known as macrophages to get to the protein in the retained fluid and break it down.

So in fact any type of fluid retention can start a vicious circle leading to worse fluid retention.

All parts of your body are drained by your lymphatic system, and Dr Casley-Smith points out that diseases of almost every organ can be caused or greatly worsened by congestion of the lymphatic system. The worst type of damage associated with protein-related inflammation is known as autoimmune attack, in which your white blood cells attack, for instance, your body's own joint tissue, nerve cells or thyroid gland. These attacks occur when your tissues begin to appear abnormal, as if they belong not to your body but to a foreign invader which must be destroyed for your body's safety. It is the presence of excess proteins in the tissue spaces that makes the tissues appear abnormal. Bacteria and other invaders are also made from proteins, and your body's immune system may not be able to tell the difference.

Lung and eye problems

When the lymphatic drainage of your lungs is impaired, chronic bronchitis and emphysema – a disease which progressively destroys the lungs' oxygen-absorbing mechanisms – may result from the associated long-term inflammation and fibrosis. Even your eyes can suffer from fluid retention. The disease known as macular degeneration – a common cause of blindness – is associated with pools of excess protein and blood leakage from capillaries behind the retina.

Stretching breaks vital contacts

One very damaging result of fluid retention is the 'stretching' effect of excess fluid on your tissue spaces. The more these spaces become engorged with fluid, the further away your cells become from their source of vital oxygen and nutrients and from each other. Even minor fluid retention can break the cell-to-cell contacts which assist the passage of oxygen from your capillaries to the part of the cell where it is needed.

As yet, we know very little about the effects this can have on your body. We know that when cells are starved of oxygen wounds fail to heal properly, but what about nutrients? When the nutrients in your tissue spaces are diluted by too much fluid, are your cells able to absorb enough of them? What if you are eating a diet that is only just adequate? Will you start to show signs of nutritional deficiencies as the nutrients fail to filter through to your cells in large enough amounts?

A possible cancer risk

It is scientifically well established that, when your tissue spaces become oversaturated with fluid, they also become much more

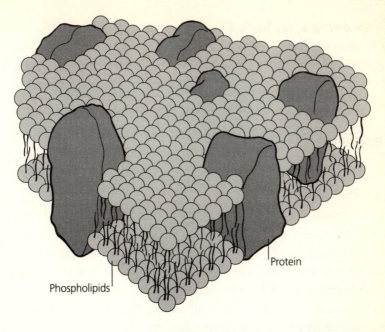

Phospholipids

Protein

Cell membrane

permeable to all kinds of possibly toxic particles which they would not normally absorb. As harmful substances such as free radicals come into contact with your cells they can rupture the delicate membrane which covers them, damaging the cell and allowing genetic material to leak out.

As explained by Dr Nadya Coates in her book *A Matter of Life*, it is a law of life that every piece of genetic material 'wants' to become a cell and to become a nucleus, but in this event it would do so without the full genetic information required for a cell to reach proper maturity. Cancer starts when an abnormal, immature cell 'born' in this way begins to reproduce wildly. Normally your immune system will seek out and destroy abnormal cells, but don't forget the various types of disruption which fluid retention and fibrosis bring to the affected areas, such as reduction of the oxygen supply and blockage of the passage of macrophages. It may one day be discovered that the efficiency of the immune system in destroying cancer cells is reduced under these conditions.

Improving Lymphatic Congestion

Once again, don't be daunted by this information. It is only included to help you take seriously the kind of lifestyle changes which will help prevent health problems or worse fluid retention in later life.

Movement

To keep the lymphatic system functioning healthily, wherever possible avoid remaining still for many hours, for example watching TV.

If you suffer an injury don't let the pain keep you immobile, since the damage in that area will make it particularly susceptible to fluid retention which will worsen the pain. You don't need to move broken bones, but if you have a broken arm, for instance, you could rotate your head and shoulder a little from time to time, stretch the rest of your body and massage under your armpit. Even small, gentle movements like this will help to prevent fluid retention.

If you suffer from any type of paralysis, regular massage will become all the more important. ME (chronic fatigue syndrome) patients may well find that getting someone to massage them every day may help some of the soreness that bed-bound sufferers often experience and which can be due to fluid build-up.

Choose flavonoids, not diuretics

The one thing which doctors should not do is treat high-protein type fluid retention with diuretic drugs, which will only dehydrate your tissues temporarily. The protein causing the fluid retention will not be removed by the drugs but will remain in your tissues and quickly attract fluid back into them. The dehydration will also constipate you, make you retain sodium and so aggravate your fluid retention. French kidney specialist Dr G. Lagrue, whose work is mentioned in other chapters of this book, describes a type of fluid retention caused by laxative and diuretic abuse.

There is another medical treatment for high-protein type fluid retention which is used by lymphologists in Australia, Germany and

More Facts about Your Capillaries

Your capillary network extends to almost every tissue of your body. Each capillary is about 1 mm long, and none of the cells in your body should be more than 0.1 mm away from a capillary. Capillaries are so tiny they can hardly be seen with the naked eye. The capillary itself is a tube whose walls are made up of flat cells one layer thick. These, known as endothelial cells, fit together with narrow, water-filled gaps or 'pores' between them. On the other side of the capillary wall is the tissue fluid, the watery fluid in your tissue spaces which bathes each cell of your body's tissues.

Oxygen and fat-soluble nutrients (nutrients which can dissolve in oil but not in water) pass from your blood through the endothelial cells to get to your tissue fluid. Water, glucose and other water-soluble nutrients pass through the water-filled pores. Once in the tissue fluid, these substances can be taken up as needed by your cells. Waste products such as carbon dioxide which are released from your cells also pass into your tissue fluid, and from here can pass into your capillaries ready for processing or elimination.

The walls of a vein, showing how the cells which it is made from are arranged. In a capillary, fluid escapes through the 'seams' between the cells.

Lymph Drainage Massage

Correct massage can improve the flow of lymph. The lymph must be worked from the outer parts of the body towards the centre, but first start at the centre to create a reservoir into which the outer (peripheral) collecting lymphatics can drain. Then gradually extend the area of massage towards the peripheral parts of the body, always working towards the centre. Some popular books suggest using a dry brush on the skin, but this is harsh on the skin and it is not known whether it provides enough stimulation to help 'pump' the lymph along. Also, some of these books wrongly state that the brush strokes should be in an outward direction rather than vice versa.

The neck, tummy, groin and armpit areas are important starting points for massage.

Lymphologists recommend that athletes and dancers should practise lymphatic drainage massage when they get mild injuries. A minute spent in emptying the lymph nodes in the groin can reduce pain in a sprained ankle and improve its mobility, which is limited both by the fluid which collects in the injured area and by the pain it causes.

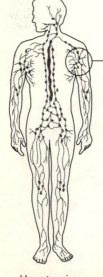

Nodes
Massage these areas first, then slowly working towards the outside of the body. Stroke in the direction of the heart.

How to give yourself a Lymphatic Drainage Massage

Italy. It consists of the flavonoids quercetin and rutin together with the plant extract coumarin. Chapter 8 describes these substances and their effects in detail. As mentioned in Chapter 6, flavonoids are important nutrients in fruits and vegetables which help to keep blood vessels strong and prevent them leaking. But Dr Casley-Smith has also carried out some fascinating research which shows that given in very high doses, they can encourage the proliferation of the white blood cells known as macrophages, which gather in parts of the body affected by high-protein type fluid retention and split the accumulated protein into small fragments. Once broken down into amino acids, the proteins are much more easily able to pass back through the capillary walls and back into the bloodstream.

If you suffer from varicose veins, you may be interested to know that one of the above-mentioned nutrients, rutin, can be used to repair damage to elastin and collagen in the walls of your veins. We mentioned in Chapter 6 that the herb gotu kola can also help varicose veins. Since herbs are plants which often contain the same flavonoids as foods, but perhaps in higher concentrations, it may be that many herbs work not by having a medicinal effect but by correcting long-term nutritional deficiencies.

Fluid Retention Caused by Vitamin and Mineral Deficiencies

It is perfectly possible to have symptoms of vitamin or mineral deficiencies even if you eat a healthy, nourishing, well-balanced diet.

Would you know if you had a nutritional deficiency? Not necessarily. A lot of the symptoms of vitamin and mineral deficiencies, for example, are things we easily take for granted:

- bad skin
- getting tired easily
- not sleeping well
- mood swings
- bad nerves
- period pains

As already explained, fluid retention can be a sign of protein deficiency, but good fluid balance also depends on adequate amounts of a lot of substances known collectively as micronutrients: vitamins, minerals, essential fatty acids, flavonoids and so on. This chapter looks at some of the ways in which these nutrients can affect your fluid balance, how nutritional deficiencies occur, and how their presence can be identified.

Case Study: Barbara

Barbara consulted me when she was seven months pregnant. She was twenty-three and a vegetarian, and it was her first baby. She came somewhat reluctantly, at the instigation of her mother-in-law. Barbara's appetite was so poor that she ate foods only for their taste, not from hunger. While the rest of the family had a complete meal, she might pick at a piece of cheesecake.

Barbara was badly anaemic. Her haemoglobin levels had been progressively dropping since the early stages of pregnancy, despite her being prescribed increasing doses of iron. By the time she consulted me her skin was extremely pale and the anaemia was causing severe fluid retention, particularly in her legs. The extra fluid was in turn pushing her blood pressure sky-high, and both mother and baby were at risk. Barbara agreed to see me because her doctor wanted to keep her in hospital in order to give her iron injections. She had refused this, and was desperately seeking alternatives.

The foods Barbara did eat included a lot of fat, white bread, chocolate, crisps and biscuits. She had received counselling about iron-rich foods from a hospital dietician, but couldn't follow the advice because she had no appetite.

She told me that she suffered from permanent sores inside her nose, and that during the first three months of her pregnancy she had felt nauseous twenty-four hours a day. In my opinion, these symptoms plus the anaemia and fluid retention pointed to severe zinc deficiency. Her diet excluded meat and fish, from which most people get their zinc, and was also lacking in wholegrains, which are a vegetarian source of zinc. To make matters worse, iron supplements can interfere with the absorption of zinc from food – yet her doctor was prescribing very large amounts of iron.

After asking her to obtain her doctor's permission to stop the iron supplements I gave her multivitamins and minerals plus zinc, together with some counselling along the lines of the Waterfall Diet. To her doctor's amazement, Barbara's haemoglobin levels started to rise within days. She went on to produce a healthy baby.

Nutritional Deficiency Questionnaire

• Do you find it hard to grip pens, cutlery or tools?
• Have you noticed a loss of sensation in your fingertips?
• Do you accidentally drop and break things much more than you used to?
• Do you ever suffer from painful leg cramps at night?
• If you are a woman, do you gain several pounds before your periods or experience a swollen tummy?
• If you are a woman who has reached the menopause, have you developed painful knots on the sides of your finger joints?
• Do you get numbness or tingling in your hands?
• Do your hands often 'go to sleep' in bed at night?
• Do you eat fresh fruit and vegetables less than once a day?
• Do you normally eat white bread rather than wholemeal?
• Do you put sugar in tea or coffee?
• Weight for weight, do you consume as much sugary food (e.g. sweets, chocolate, cakes, biscuits, jam, honey, syrup, ice cream, sugary cereals, desserts and sweet drinks) as other foods – or perhaps even more?
• Do you eat fried or fatty food such as burgers, sausages or pastry every day?
• Has there ever been a time in your life when you ate an extremely poor diet for several months or even years?

If you have answered yes to six or more of the above questions, your fluid retention could be due to nutritional deficiencies.

B6 – an Exciting Discovery

Pyridoxine, or vitamin B6, was isolated in 1938. It seems incredible that we have known about this important nutrient for such a short time, and even more incredible that only in 1952 was the discovery made that it is essential for human life. Some babies in the USA developed convulsions after consuming an excessively heated commercial milk formula; the cause was found to be deficiency of vitamin B6, which is destroyed by heat. A fascinating account of this discovery is given in a book published in 1973, *Vitamin B6: The Doctor's Report,* by Dr John Ellis from Texas.

Dr Ellis developed a strong interest in vitamin B6 in 1961, and spent the next nine years conducting clinical studies in its thera-peutic use. Around this time doctors were finding that more and more ailments responded to vitamin B6 therapy, which implied that they had been brought on by a deficiency of this vitamin. These conditions included seizures in mentally retarded children, neuritis associated with the use of anti-TB drugs, nausea from cancer radiotherapy treatments, anaemia which did not respond to the usual therapies, and sunburn after very little exposure to the sun. In addition, Dr Ellis found that vitamin B6 deficiency could cause severe fluid retention.

The diet that worked

His interest began when he started to investigate diet and nutri-tion after heart disease had killed several of his patients. After reading about the Morrison diet, recommended in the *Journal of the American Medical Association,* he began prescribing it to his patients. The diet advocated lean instead of fatty meat, increased consumption of fruit and vegetables, and the use of vegetable oils instead of animal fats.

Many of his patients had complained of tingling sensations, cramps and spasms but the diet appeared to relieve these symptoms. Some patients whose hands were puffy (a sign of fluid retention) and could not bend their fingers very well lost both the puffiness and several pounds in weight, and became able to bend their fingers easily, within a few weeks and without cutting down on their calorie intake. One of the patients had cured pains in his knees by eating pecan nuts every day, and said that he too had lost stiffness in his fingers and now had a stronger grip. The doctor added pecan nuts to the Morrison diet, and got even better results.

Putting two and two together

At this point Dr Ellis didn't know *why* the diet was causing these improvements, but he did know that it was much richer in B vitamins than what his patients had previously been eating. He persuaded some of them to try vitamin B injections for the tingling and pains in their hands, and he found this treatment to be just as successful as the new diet. Putting two and two together, he concluded that:

- the numbness, tingling, pains, puffiness and gripping problems were caused by fluid retention
- the fluid retention was a symptom of B vitamin deficiency.

No doctor had ever reported this before.

The proof

Excited at his findings, Ellis wondered which specific B vitamin his patients most lacked. It could not be B1 because this deficiency caused tremors of the tongue. B2 deficiency led to little sores in the corners of the mouth. B3 deficiency gave rise to dermatitis. His patients did not have any of these symptoms.

No medical reports had yet suggested that B6 deficiency could occur in adults, but Dr Ellis wondered what the symptoms would be if it did. He decided to try injecting plain vitamin B6 into his patients, knowing that, medically speaking, he was in completely uncharted territory. As he waited for the results, he knew he could be on the threshold of a tremendous discovery. Fluid retention was one of the most baffling problems facing his medical colleagues.

Seeing the first patient return to his surgery after four days, having lost so much excess fluid that her shoes were now several sizes too big for her, was the greatest thrill Dr Ellis had experienced in his entire medical career.

What Are the Symptoms of Vitamin B6 Deficiency?

While official textbooks are slow in catching up with John Ellis' observational studies on his patients, they do now recognize that vitamin B6 deficiency can occur in adults, particularly in

- those on anti-TB medications
- those who drink a lot of alcohol
- up to 20 per cent of women who take the contraceptive pill.

They also recognize that, because vitamin B6 deficiency can increase the excretion of a chemical known as oxalate in the urine, it may contribute to kidney stones. Pregnancy, heart failure and radiation exposure are also recognized as leading to higher requirements for B6. Experimental B6 deprivation has resulted in symptoms of irritability, weakness, insomnia and poor coordination, say the official books. Nowhere is there any reference to fluid retention. Yet without vitamin B6 important amino acids cannot be synthesized from other amino acids; the vital brain messenger chemicals serotonin, noradrenaline and histamine cannot be made from the amino acids tryptophan, tyrosine and histidine. Vitamin B3 cannot be made from the amino acid tryptophan. Perhaps most important of all, vitamin B6 assists in the transport of amino acids from the intestine across the gut wall and in the blood. Without this transport, a protein deficiency could develop.

But lymph expert Dr John Casley-Smith, whose work was mentioned in Chapter 7, does have something to say about fluid retention and the B vitamins. He points out that a diet lacking these nutrients causes the gaps between cells lining the blood capillaries to open up, allowing protein to escape into the tissue space, where it attracts excess fluid. And in experiments, rats deprived of all B vitamins for 42 days develop leaks in their lymphatic vessels. Giving them vitamins B5 or B6, or flavonoids (see below), prevents this. Diets lacking in flavonoids, or in vitamin C, can make capillaries even more leaky, and advanced vitamin C deficiency – the condition known as scurvy – leads to leakage of whole blood, not just fluid, out of the capillaries, resulting in little red blood marks under the skin.

Premenstrual Syndrome

Millions of women experience the discomfort of swollen, painful breasts and bloated tummies around the time of their period.

These symptoms are due to fluid retention. If you suffer from them, you will probably have noticed that your body weight goes down soon after your period starts.

B6 and magnesium deficiency

Writing in the *Journal of Reproductive Medicine*, nutrition specialist Dr Guy Abrahams is sure that premenstrual fluid retention is caused by temporary deficiencies of vitamin B6 and the mineral magnesium, brought on by the extra nutritional demands of hormonal changes. In a woman's monthly cycle oestrogen levels steadily increase until ovulation, after which she makes increased amounts of progesterone while her liver breaks down the excess oestrogen. All these processes make heavy use of many nutrients. Since vitamin B6 plays an especially important role it risks getting depleted at certain times.

B6 deficiency not only promotes fluid retention by weakening the capillary walls but can also affect your body's excretion of sodium. Both B6 and the mineral magnesium (see below) are required for the production of dopamine, a hormone which, by counteracting the effects of the sodium-retaining hormone aldosterone (see Chapter 4) would normally encourage your body to excrete sodium and water. Dr Abrahams quotes research which has found that levels of dopamine are low in women who retain fluid premenstrually.

Finally, vitamin B6 and magnesium (among other nutrients) are needed for the production of beneficial prostaglandins, which are also involved in controlling the body's fluid balance. There will be more about this on p. 113.

Research studies reporting that giving B6 supplements to women with premenstrual syndrome can prevent their symptoms have been published in the *Journal of International Medical Research* in 1985, the *Journal of Reproductive Medicine* in 1987, the *Lancet* in 1988 and the *British Medical Journal* in 1999, among others. But success using this approach has been variable, which is not surprising.

This book has shown that the causes of even such an apparently straightforward symptom as fluid retention can be complex and varied. Conducting research which assumes that all women with premenstrual fluid retention are suffering from the same nutritional deficiency and giving them the same vitamin supplement may, if the results of all these studies are merged, show roughly how many cases are due to vitamin B6 deficiency and how many are not. But it does not help doctors to decide which of the women consulting them should be given the supplements.

Magnesium

Several hundred enzyme reactions in the human body depend on magnesium, yet when doctors in the UK test for nutritional deficiencies, they find magnesium (and zinc and selenium) are lacking more frequently than any other minerals.

What are you eating?

Most people eat a diet low in magnesium-rich foods such as wholemeal bread, oatmeal, nuts, sesame seeds and dark green leafy vegetables. Did you know, for instance, that white flour contains only one-third as much magnesium as wholemeal flour? To make matters worse, excessive protein in your diet, especially dairy produce, can render magnesium less easily taken up by your body because of the high phosphorus and calcium content. So your potential magnesium deficiency is further aggravated.

Cut coffee and stress

Coffee consumption increases the excretion of magnesium and other minerals. Magnesium can also be depleted by:

- chronic diarrhoea
- overuse of enemas or laxatives
- the contraceptive pill
- one of the biggest drains on magnesium is stress.

A little-known fact is that stress hormones such as adrenaline and cortisol lower your body's magnesium levels too. According to specialist researchers, all stress, whether exertion, heat, cold, trauma, pain, anxiety, excitement or even asthma attacks, can have this effect and so increase your need for magnesium. This important subject was extensively reviewed in 1994 in the prestigious *Journal of the American College of Nutrition*.

The link with potassium

Since magnesium is needed for so many enzymes in your body, it is involved in fluid balance in many ways. For instance, it is known to biochemists that magnesium and the mineral potassium work so closely together in the body's cells that doctors cannot improve low potassium levels in their heart patients, for example, or in patients on potent diuretic drugs, unless they first correct any magnesium deficiency.

The journal *Archives of Internal Medicine* reports that 38–42 per cent of such patients have magnesium deficiency, and the *American Journal of Medicine* goes even further, stating that 'Hypomagnesemia [magnesium deficiency] is probably the most underdiagnosed electrolyte deficiency in current medical practice.' (See Chapter 4 if you need to be reminded about electrolytes, and how the balance between sodium and potassium inside and outside your body's cells decides how much water is excreted by your kidneys.) If you are retaining fluid because you are losing too much potassium it may be due to magnesium deficiency, and can be helped by eating more magnesium-rich foods – as in the Waterfall Diet – and if necessary also taking magnesium supplements.

B6 to the rescue

Vitamin B6 helps to get magnesium across the cell membrane and into your cells. In one research study published in the *Annals of Clinical Laboratory Science*, a group of nine women were found to have low levels of magnesium in their red blood cells (magnesium deficiency shows up more quickly in the red blood cells than it does in the blood plasma where it is usually measured!). After receiving 100 mg of vitamin B6 twice a day these levels rose significantly, and doubled after four weeks of treatment. If we make the reasonable assumption that red blood cells will only absorb as much magnesium as they need, this research would suggest that these women's red cells were previously not absorbing enough magnesium, due to a lack of vitamin B6.

Yet more effects of magnesium deficiency

It has already been mentioned that a magnesium (and vitamin B6) deficiency results in reduced levels of the hormone dopamine, which helps to counteract the sodium-retention hormone aldosterone. Research carried out in the Department of Diabetes at the City of Hope Medical Center in Duarte, California, has found that a magnesium deficiency is also associated with higher levels of aldosterone. So magnesium deficiency is a double candidate for promoting fluid retention.

The formerly mysterious fluid retention and associated high blood pressure which sometimes occurs in pregnancy is now becoming recognized and treated as a magnesium deficiency condition, since magnesium infusions have proved to be a more effective treatment than drugs. It is very unfortunate for other types of patients who are in great need of magnesium that their doctors have perhaps not read the articles in medical journals which might have resulted in more effective treatments, using magnesium instead.

Anaemia

The most common nutritional deficiency disease in the Western world is anaemia – a condition in which the red blood cells are not able to absorb enough oxygen.

Iron deficiency anaemia

Normally assumed to be due to iron deficiency, most anaemia is treated with iron supplements and an iron-rich diet of red meat, liver and green vegetables. Only recently have dieticians been made aware of research indicating that one cause of iron deficiency can be a lack of vitamin C-rich foods eaten as part of meals (iron is much better absorbed from plant foods in the presence of larger amounts of vitamin C).

Anaemia can cause fluid retention in two ways. First, severe anaemia seems to encourage sodium retention by the kidneys. As we know, this leads to fluid retention. Second, severe anaemia which goes on for too long can damage the heart. The heart works harder and harder as it tries to get the blood around to the lungs again as quickly as possible in order to pick up more oxygen. Eventually it starts to fail and has difficulty pumping blood at all. Due to the low fluid pressure in the kidneys, severe fluid retention develops.

Other types of anaemia

While iron deficiency anaemia is the most common type, deficiencies of the following can cause it too:

- folic acid
- vitamin B2
- vitamin B6 (sometimes associated with taking the contraceptive pill)
- vitamin B12
- vitamin C
- vitamin E
- copper
- zinc
- protein

Lack of these nutrients causes anaemia by impairing the formation of healthy red blood cells.

Macrocytic anaemia, characterized by reduced numbers of red blood cells, which become abnormally large and malformed, is caused by vitamin B12 and folic acid deficiencies. Pernicious anaemia, caused by a failure to absorb vitamin B12, is a type of macrocytic anaemia.

Sickle cell anaemia is due to abnormal haemoglobin (the oxygen-carrying part of the red blood cell), whch results in distorted and fragile red blood cells. Plasma levels of vitamin B6 can be abnormally low in sufferers. Research reported in the *American Journal of Clinical Nutrition* in 1984 suggests that people with this illness can greatly benefit from supplementation with 100 mg of vitamin B6 per day. The supplements can increase both the number of red blood cells and their haemoglobin levels. This suggests that sickle cell patients have much higher vitamin B6 needs than the rest of the population.

Essential Polyunsaturated Oils

Both magnesium and vitamin B6 are among the nutrients which help to turn the essential polyunsaturated oils in your diet into prostaglandins. As we saw in Chapter 7, prostaglandins are hormone-like, locally-acting substances involved in the control of your body fluid levels, blood pressure and many other functions. 'Locally acting' means that they may cause fluid retention in one of your joints, for example, while leaving the rest of your body unaffected. Prostaglandins are produced within the phospholipids (fatty compounds which contain phosphate) making up your cell membranes – the delicate protective sheath which surrounds each cell. Apart from magnesium and vitamin B6, the other important nutrients involved in the production of prostaglandins are zinc, biotin, selenium, iron and vitamins B3, C and E.

Balancing your prostaglandins

Those made from arachidonic acid can promote fluid retention by increasing the leakiness of your blood capillaries and encouraging inflammation such as skin rashes or pain and swelling in joints. One of the jobs of the beneficial Series 1 and 3 types is to prevent the release of excessive amounts of arachidonic acid from your cell membranes. This prevents unnecessary amounts of the arachidonic acid prostaglandins from being made.

It is not difficult to keep down your levels of arachidonic acid (Series 2) prostaglandins. Animal fat, found in meat, dairy products and eggs, is the only source of arachidonic acid in food, so if you avoid these foods you may be able to reduce fluid retention in

HOW OILS ARE BROKEN DOWN TO PROSTAGLANDINS

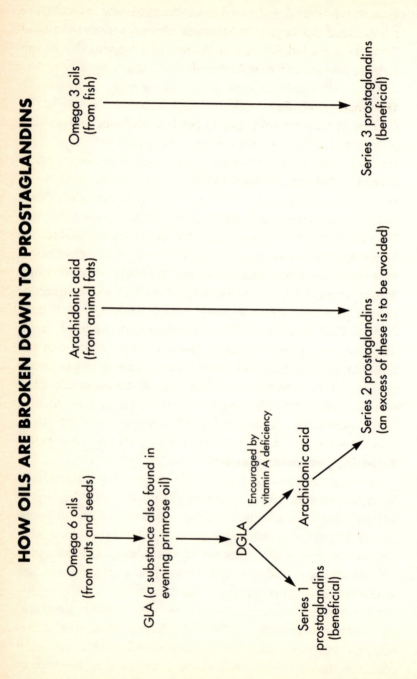

your skin or joints, which in turn causes pain and inflammation as described in Chapter 7. Although your body does need small amounts of arachidonic acid, it can satisfy these needs by synthesizing it from other fats and oils.

The value of oily fish

Correcting your vitamin and mineral deficiencies will in time bring about the enzyme repairs necessary to keep your prostaglandins in the right balance. In the meantime you can help control the release of arachidonic acid from your cell membranes by regularly eating the oily fish such as salmon, sardines, pilchards, herrings and mackerel. A portion of one of these every few days will help you make much larger amounts of beneficial Series 3 prostaglandins. In fact, this could be the reason why some women with premenstrual fluid retention derive so much benefit from eating a diet rich in these fish. The fish oils are acting as a medicine, altering the women's body chemistry.

Dr William Rea, Professor of Environmental Medicine at the University of Surrey in England, points out that excessive amounts of arachidonic acid prostaglandins are found in people suffering from a wide variety of chronic illnesses, including asthma and arthritis as well as premenstrual syndrome. Nutritional experts who specialize in this field are blaming this on deficiencies of the vitamins and minerals which help to make the beneficial prostaglandins which control arachidonic acid.

To supplement or not?

Fish oil supplements are not very strong and contain only a fraction of the active nutrient (known as EPA) found in oily fish themselves. Supplements of evening primrose oil, blackcurrant seed oil and borage oil can also be used to alleviate premenstrual syndrome and diseases involving inflammation. The active ingredient in these supplements is known as GLA. It can be turned either into beneficial Series 1 prostaglandins, or into much less desirable arachidonic acid. Professor Rea warns that vitamin A deficiency may encourage the latter. Perhaps it would be a good idea for vitamin manufacturers to put some vitamin A (with zinc, which is often deficient and helps the body to use this vitamin) in their evening primrose oil products. Research using evening primrose oil to treat eczema, arthritis and PMS might then produce more consistently successful results in clinical trials.

Flavonoids

As explained in Chapter 7, if the walls of your blood capillaries are weakened, they can leak excess fluid and protein from your blood into your tissue spaces, thus causing fluid retention. This weakness of the capillaries is referred to as capillary fragility. As long ago as the 1930s it was discovered that one particular type of nutritional deficiency was especially likely to cause capillary fragility. The nutrients concerned are known as flavonoids (or sometimes by the more old-fashioned term 'bioflavonoids'). These substances are powerful antioxidants found in fruit and vegetables, and are responsible for some of their colours such as the red or blue of grape and berry skins. Apart from their antioxidant activity, flavonoids are known for their ability to prevent and treat bruising, varicose veins, bleeding gums and nosebleeds. They may also be useful in the treatment of heavy menstrual bleeding where no apparent cause is found on medical investigation. A third beneficial effect of the flavonoids quercetin, rutin, curcumin, silymarin and green tea polyphenols is their reputed anti-inflammatory effect, which works in a similar way to aspirin.

It is often said that flavonoids work by 'strengthening' the capillaries (see p. 85) and that this is why they improve the circulation, eyesight and intellect. This implies that the foods containing them need only be consumed – like a kind of medicine – if you have circulatory problems. In fact flavonoids can only *normalize* capillaries and circulation which have been made leaky by insufficient fruit and vegetables in the diet.

Lemons (outer skin and white pith), and the central white core of all citrus fruit, are a particularly rich source of flavonoids. The white pith of green peppers is also good, as is the skin of colourful

Benefits of Some Common Flavonoids

Name	Found in	Effects
Anthocyanidins	Blue pigments (may appear red under some conditions) found in berry skins, especially bilberries	Beneficial effects on eyesight and circulation, and some antibacterial action
Hesperidin	Citrus pith	Improves abnormal capillary fragility. Anti-allergic: helps to minimize the effects of histamine
Myricetin	Ginkgo biloba	Helps to prevent free radical damage to nerve cells
Nobiletin	Citrus fruits	Has anti-inflammatory action and assists detoxification
Proanthocyanidins (also known as pycnogenols)	Pine bark, tea, peanut skins, cranberries, grape seeds and skins	Their antioxidant potency (particularly the varieties found in grape seeds) is reputedly twenty times greater than that of vitamin E
Quercetin	Apple peel, onions, tea, ginkgo biloba and cabbage. Can also be synthesized by intestinal bacteria from rutin (see below)	Structurally related to the anti-allergic drug disodium chromoglycate, quercetin may help allergy-related problems such as hay fever, asthma and eczema. It also decreases the synthesis of pro-inflammatory prostaglandins. Research has shown that it helps prevent eye cataracts which can lead to blindness
Rutin	Buckwheat and buckwheat tea	Helps in the treatment of high blood pressure, bruising and haemorrhages under the skin, including redness due to radiation. Has been used in the treatment of varicose veins
Silybin	The herb milk thistle and its extract silymarin	Silymarin is a well-researched liver protective and regenerative substance which also protects cell membranes against damage by toxins

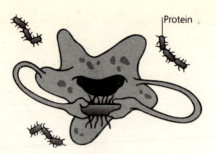

A macrophage

berries and grapes. Some herbs such as ginkgo biloba (see p. 122) are taken partly for the action of their flavonoids.

Rutin, quercetin and coumarin

Dr John Casley-Smith has carried out extensive research with the flavonoids rutin and quercetin and the related substance coumarin. He has found that not only can leaky capillaries repair themselves when these substances are consumed, but the number of white blood cells known as macrophages increases in areas where excess protein has leaked into the tissue spaces. The macrophages produce enzymes which split the proteins into fragments that can then be reabsorbed by the blood capillaries. Once the excess protein has been removed the often painful inflammation caused by it ceases, and the excess fluid which inevitably accompanies it in the tissue spaces drains away in the blood or lymph.

Natural medicine practitioners have always treated diseases involving inflammation, such as arthritis and skin rashes, with 'cleansing' diets of fruit and vegetables and their juices. Large amounts of flavonoids can be consumed in such diets, and may well account for the many success stories. Having endured scorn for many decades from other areas of the medical profession who call their work 'unproven', natural medicine practitioners are delighted that so much modern research is confirming the value of their nutritional treatments.

As we saw in Chapter 7, capillary walls can also be weakened by a vitamin C deficiency, and lymphology experts have found

that vitamin C supplements can also help to reduce high
type fluid retention.

Coumarin, a substance related to flavonoids, gives hay its char-
acteristic sweet smell and is found in clover flowers, red wine,
orange pith, red peppers, parsley, celery, horse chestnuts and
many other foods and herbs. It is also effective against high-
protein type fluid retention when applied as a cream, for instance
to an arthritic joint. Although it appears to be little used outside
Germany and Switzerland, your doctor should be able to
prescribe it for you if your pharmacist can track down a source
(see below).

Quercetin and rutin may also have an anti-allergy effect. As
already mentioned, allergic reactions usually involve the release of
histamine which increases the leakiness of blood capillaries, thus
encouraging fluid retention. Coumarin and several flavonoids can
inhibit histamine release.

Some Common Foods and Herbs Which Contain Coumarin

Alfalfa	Celery	Meadowsweet
Angelica	Chamomile flowers	Nettle
Aniseed	Fenugreek seeds	Parsley
Asafoetida	Horse-chestnut extract	Red clover flowers
Bitter lettuce (leaf and	Horseradish root	Siberian ginseng
sap)	King's clover flowers	Wild lettuce
Boldo	Liquorice root	Woodruff
Cayenne (chilli pepper)		

Coumarin is better absorbed through the skin than by mouth. Make yourself the
following special remedies

Coumarin Bath Recipe

Clover can be found growing wherever there is grass: meadows, heaths, road-
sides and so on. Pick a large bag of clover flowers and allow the flowers to dry in
the sun. Coumarin levels in clover flowers rise as a result of wilting and drying. Tie
up a handful of the flowers in a piece of muslin or nappy liner (the latter can be
stapled together to make a kind of envelope) and soak this in your bathwater
before having a bath.

Coumarin Tea

Pour some boiling water on to a few dried clover flowers and drink as a tea.
Flavour with other ingredients too if you wish, such as chamomile, which also
contains coumarin.

...etention, if your arthritis, eczema, ...problems are caused by allergy you may ...oid-rich foods (see the table on p. 137) or ...xtractor to turn them into drinks, enabling ...more of them.

Treating ... oedema with coumarin

One of the biggest challenges to lymphologists is the high-protein type fluid retention known as lymphoedema, which occurs when the lymphatic system becomes obstructed. For instance the type of mastectomy operation which removes the under-arm lymph nodes as well as a woman's breast is a big cause of lymphoedema in the affected arm. Removal of the lymph nodes in the groin can make a leg swell up to twice its normal diameter.

Dr Casley-Smith uses pharmaceutical coumarin to treat these cases, but unless a doctor has read the journals in which coumarin research has been reported, he will normally advise nothing but compression bandages, raising the affected limb, exercise and perhaps massage. In one coumarin trial, one group of mastectomy patients who had had their under-arm lymph nodes removed were given compression bandages and advised to exercise their arms and keep them raised as much as possible, while a second group was also given daily doses of coumarin. The patients' arm circumference was then measured at regular intervals. In the first group, average arm circumference steadily increased as time went by, while in the second group there was a slow but steady reduction amounting to 3.3 mm every ten months. The second group also suffered less from bursting pains, cramps, tension in the limb and secondary acute inflammation.

If you suffer from lymphoedema, you should be able to get coumarin on prescription. In the UK, ask your doctor to prescribe Lodema®. Your pharmacist will be able to track down a UK supplier. If you live elsewhere or have any problems obtaining Lodema, see Useful Addresses on p. 202.

Safety

Don't worry – quercetin and rutin are not harmful. Even when the individual flavonoids are extracted and sold as dietary supplements, they have not been found to cause any toxicity problems in clinical trials which use them in very high doses.

Coumarin too is generally safe, although not yet available in concentrated form over the counter in the UK. It has sometimes mistakenly been stigmatized as a human liver toxin, but this is inaccurate. It is a liver toxin for certain species of animals, but humans, and animals with a similar metabolism to humans, are not normally harmed by it. Occasional (one in 300–400) users of medically prescribed pharmaceutical coumarin may develop 'coumarin hepatitis' after some months of use. This is a reversible condition and not considered dangerous. Doctors who are experienced in prescribing pharmaceutical coumarin advise their patients to come back if they feel 'really unwell'. They are then given liver function tests and coumarin is stopped if the tests show there is a problem. The liver then returns to normal.

Coumarin is not the same substance as the blood-thinning drug warfarin, although confusion often arises between the two. Whilst sometimes also referred to as coumarin, warfarin in fact consists of dicoumarin – a derivative of coumarin.

Varicose Veins: A Type of Fluid Retention Caused by Flavonoid Deficiency?

An unsightly problem in which the veins in the legs swell and the legs themselves retain fluid, varicose veins are caused by what is known as chronic venous insufficiency – high pressure in the leg veins because the blood there has difficulty in overcoming the effects of gravity as it returns to the heart. The standard treatment is compression therapy and keeping the legs raised. Surgery may eventually be used to strip out the offending veins if the patient complains too much!

How can doctors have missed the 1996 article in the world-famous medical journal the *Lancet* reporting that the herb horse chestnut – a rich source of a coumarin-like compound (see p. 119) –

reduced fluid retention in patients with this condition almost as effectively as compression therapy? But unlike compression therapy, coumarin corrected the cause of the problem.

The *European Journal of Clinical Pharmacology* has reported success with a treatment based on flavonoids. In a double-blind clinical trial, buckwheat tea significantly reduced fluid retention in the legs of people with chronic venous insufficiency.

Results of clinical trials like these, which apply only one of the many nutritional corrective measures which an individual patient may need to treat his or her diet-related health problems, must of necessity be limited. Who knows what results these two trials could have achieved if they had made practical use of *all* the information in this chapter?

Ginkgo Biloba as a Treatment for Chronic Fluid Retention

The herb ginkgo biloba, a rich source of flavonoids, has been subjected to numerous clinical trials to improve the circulation, especially in the brain of elderly people. French kidney specialist Dr G. Lagrue of the Henri Mondor Hospital in Créteil, France, successfully used it on fifteen women who had tested positive for leaky capillaries and high-protein type fluid retention. The most severely affected women lost 4-10 lb (1.8–4.5 kg) of fluid, and the rest had good to excellent results. This trial was published in the prestigious French medical journal *La Presse Medicale* in 1986.

For the cause of fluid retention in women Dr Lagrue proposes a theory which it is interesting to compare with Dr Abrahams' theory on PMS (see p. 108). While Dr Abrahams proposes vitamin B6 deficiency as the cause of the hormonal stimulation of the kidneys to retain sodium (and therefore water), Dr Lagrue blames a relative lack of the hormone progesterone compared with levels of oestrogen. At the same time, says Dr Lagrue, the woman's blood capillaries are too leaky. This makes protein pass into her tissue spaces, attracting water from her blood. As her blood volume is reduced, the sodium-retaining hormone aldosterone tries to increase it by making her retain sodium and therefore

water. He proposes a two-fold treatment: correcting the progesterone deficiency and treating the capillary leakiness with
flavonoids.

Although Dr Lagrue does not suggest this treatment specifically for *premenstrual* fluid retention, there is no reason why it
would not be effective. Dr Lagrue substitutes flavonoids for Dr
Abrahams' vitamin B6 treatment, but flavonoids and B vitamins
often seem to have a similar therapeutic effect on leaky blood
vessels (see p. 107). In fact Dr Casley-Smith points out that
flavonoids may be able to substitute for B vitamins in this
respect.

As far as progesterone deficiency is concerned, the treatment
normally consists of administering progestogen drugs. Unfortunately, apart from the other side-effects mentioned in Chapter 5
they can also encourage fluid retention. Dr Abrahams points out
that high levels of oestrogen in the body are often responsible for
impairing the production of progesterone, and he suggests using
liver-enhancing treatments which encourage the body to break
down excess oestrogen more efficiently. For example, although
magnesium deficiency is, as we have seen, quite common, magnesium is essential for the liver processes involved in ridding the
body of excess oestrogen. Consuming a magnesium-rich daily diet
of wholegrains, sesame seeds and steamed or stir-fried green
vegetables (as in the Waterfall Diet), together with magnesium
supplements, if necessary, would be a very sensible precaution if
you are a PMS sufferer.

How Common Are Nutritional Deficiencies?

We have referred a great deal to 'nutritional deficiences' as causes
of leaky capillaries and other problems leading to fluid retention.
But perhaps you have never really considered yourself as a potential candidate for nutritional deficiencies? Most people who eat an
average diet never really think about whether their body is getting
enough vitamins and minerals, essential polyunsaturated oils and
so on, and most have never even heard of flavonoids!

Orthodox nutritionists and doctors maintain that nutritional deficiencies are very rare in the western world, although they acknowledge that certain groups of people may be at risk: expectant mothers, dieters, the elderly, children and vegetarians.

But clinical trials published in some of the world's most eminent medical and nutritional journals have found that certain 'incurable' health problems can disappear when consumption of a particular vitamin, mineral or other nutrient is increased. What does this mean? Certainly that some people have much higher needs for these nutrients than others. If those needs are not being met, is the person in question not suffering from a nutritional deficiency?

In carrying out the research for my earlier book the *Nutritional Health Bible*, I came across hundreds of these trials published since the mid-1980s alone. Since few doctors now take much notice of clinical trials published in the 1950s and 60s, I did not include these in the book, but in those days vitamin research was in its heyday, as medical workers tried to find out whether any more so-called 'mystery' diseases like pellagra and beri-beri were really just nutritional deficiencies.

Now all this research has been largely forgotten, which is very sad for the people who could benefit from the knowledge gained. A good example is schizophrenia. Dr Abram Hoffer was a practising psychiatrist during the heyday of nutritional medicine research, was converted to the nutritional approach after the many successes he achieved with it, and is still practising now (in Canada). He is quite sure that schizophrenia is a disease caused primarily by vitamin B3 deficiency. He points out that there is no difference between schizophrenia and pellagra, the vitamin B3 deficiency disease. They are so similar that in 1940s America after it was shown that vitamin B3 could cure pellagra, psychiatric patients were given supplements of the vitamin. If they responded to it, they received a diagnosis of pellagra. If not they were labelled with schizophrenia. But *some* patients labelled with schizophrenia were subsequently given extra-large amounts of vitamin B3 – up to 50 times the normal daily intake from food – and recovered.

What Causes Nutritional Deficiencies?

There are still parts of the world where people suffer starvation and malnutrition. So how can we presume to talk about 'nutritional deficiencies' in the affluent West?

The problem here is that it is not usually a lack of food which leads to deficiency but ignorance about healthy eating. Many people have no idea of their body's nutritional needs; a recent survey I was involved in found that relatively few children nowadays are ever given a proper meal with fresh vegetables. In the UK at least, a whole generation of young people has grown up eating little other than chips, burgers, crisps and chocolate, with most of their knowledge of nutrition based on television advertisements for highly processed foods. It is impossible to prove that poor nutrition is mainly esponsible for today's overflowing doctors' surgeries and hospitals, for the escalating rates of childhood asthma, diseased arteries, cancers, mental illness, premenstrual and menopausal symptoms, infertility, skin diseases, kidney disease and diabetes. There will always be someone to say that nutrition has nothing to do with these things, but the longer they do, the greater the cost to the nation as more people take time off work due to ill health, or are prescribed hysterectomies and other operations, or drugs to control their pain or help them breathe. Healthy eating does not mean eating the occasional portion of spinach when you remember. As in the Waterfall Diet, it is about eating several portions of fruits and vegetables every day, as well as making sure that most of your bread is wholemeal, and balancing the rest of your diet too. This really will minimize your risk of getting a diet-related illness.

But the story does not end here. What about schizophrenia sufferers who did not become well until they were given vitamin B3 supplements fifty times stronger than the normal intake? Children with asthma who can come off medication if they take fifty or a hundred times the normal intake of vitamin B6 but not less? And PMS sufferers who do not lose their symptoms unless they take strong B vitamin and magnesium supplements? There are many more examples in the medical literature. These people are obviously suffering from symptoms due to a greatly increased need for certain vitamins – far more than could be obtained from diet alone.

Is Malabsorption of Nutrients the Culprit?

There is still much that we do not know or understand about the human body. I believe that these cases can only be explained by an inability to absorb vitamins or minerals normally. If an individual's failing absorption mechanisms are, for example, only absorbing 10 per cent of a particular vitamin, then by consuming 10 times the usual level, in the form of a supplement, the person can absorb an amount more adequate for his or her needs, allowing their body to repair the damage which was causing the deficiency symptoms. This is probably why so many people experience health benefits from taking dietary supplements.

Absorption mechanisms are found at several levels. The first involves your digestion. If you do not produce enough acid in your stomach (and it is said that 40 per cent of people over 60 do not), then the rest of your digestive processes may not be properly triggered. If you do not digest your food properly, it will not be broken down into small enough particles to be absorbed by the walls of your intestines and so to nourish your body.

Food allergies, harmful bacterial or yeast overgrowth, or too much poorly digested food can trigger inflammation in your intestines, and may be experienced as:

- bloating
- discomfort
- irritable bowel syndrome

As we have seen, chronic inflammation leads to fluid retention and harmful changes in the body's tissues; the delicate mechanisms for absorbing food through the intestinal walls will certainly be disrupted by any inflammation here.

Once nutrients have been absorbed into your blood, they still have to be assimilated into the cells which use them. Many do not simply pass from your blood to your cells, but require special mechanisms. Virtually nothing is known about how factors like fluid retention, virus damage, chemical toxins and pollutants, or lack of oxygen affect assimilation. It is known that your cells can be fooled by certain pollutants into believing that they are nutrients (for example your nerve cells can absorb lead instead of calcium, which causes them to malfunction). It is also known that fluid retention will dilute the nutrients in your tissue spaces as your cells attempt to absorb them and that this probably reduces assimilation, as it does with oxygen. Finally, people who suffered severe vitamin B deficiency, such as former inmates of World War II Japanese prison camps, and those who had the B3 deficiency disease pellagra in 1930s America, are known to have developed extra B vitamin needs so great that they must have had barely any assimilation ability left at all.

How do you Know if You Have Extra-large Needs for Certain Nutrients?

If you have followed the advice in this book for several months and still have some of the symptoms of nutritional deficiency listed on p. 199, it is possible that you might have extra large needs. To find out for certain you can have 'functional' tests carried out. These tests measure not the amount of a nutrient in your blood, but how well the functions in your body which depend on that nutrient are being carried out. Most functional tests are relatively new, and although a few family doctors are using them you will probably need to have them done privately through a nutritional therapist (see Useful Addresses on p. 202).

Reducing fluid retention with the Waterfall Diet is sure to help improve the uptake of oxygen and nutrients by your cells, which can only mean better health for your skin, hair, eyes, bones, hormones, brain, nerves and arteries, and more energy and vitality for *you*.

Combating Heart Disease

What most people refer to as heart disease is actually a disease of the coronary arteries which supply your heart muscle with blood.

What happens in your body? Cholesterol deposits on the coronary artery walls can eventually reduce the blood supply, leaving your heart short of oxygen. If the arteries become very narrow, angina pain occurs whenever you exert yourself. Complete oxygen starvation, as when a small clot lodges in the artery, is experienced as a heart attack (when part of the heart tissue dies) or cardiac arrest – the heart stops functioning completely.

After a heart attack, the damage tissue often leads to abnormalities in your heart's structure and reduced efficiency. As your heart struggles to keep up with its workload, it may in time start to fail – its pumping action may become unable to get blood around your body fast enough to keep all your organs supplied with enough oxygen and nutrients. This condition is known as congestive heart failure or CHF. The heart will often become enlarged as it attempts to work harder, and fluid retention can be a big problem.

People with congestive heart failure absorb less and less oxygen, and develop fatigue, a chronic dry cough, shortness of breath and a bluish tinge to the lips.

Congestive heart failure can also develop without any previous damage to your heart, if your heart's workload becomes abnormally large for too long. Severe anaemia, for example, when the red blood cells are not able to absorb enough oxygen from the lungs, forces the heart to pump much harder as it attempts to get the blood around to the lungs again as quickly as possible. Other conditions which can damage the heart or increase its workload and so possibly lead to enlarged heart and CHF include:

- Alcoholism
- Severe vitamin B1 deficiency
- Untreated high blood pressure
- Thyroid abnormalities
- The lung diseases emphysema, asthma and chronic bronchitis
- Severe fluid retention
- Severe overweight

Standard medical treatments for CHF are restricted to treating the symptoms: diuretic drugs (see Chapter 5) to reduce the fluid retention, other drugs to dilate your blood vessels, slow your heart rate and help it to pump, and advice to avoid excitement and exertion. Some doctors will also prescribe a low-salt diet. But research shows that a great deal more can be done for this life-threatening illness.

A combination of treatments

Natural treatments for CHF are used in addition to conventional treatments, and centre around the causes.

- Does the patient have a long-standing vitamin B6 deficiency or food allergy which caused the original fluid retention?
- What about magnesium deficiency, associated with asthma and high blood pressure?
- Was he/she very deficient in flavonoids, and so developed leaky capillaries and inflammation in the lungs after breathing in fumes or smoke, possibly progressing to chronic bronchitis and emphysema?

If you or a relative are determined to do your very best to combat this illness, the Waterfall Diet will give you a very good start, since it is so rich in all the right nutrients. For the same reason it will help to reduce cholesterol levels and some people find that problems like angina and high blood pressure start to disappear.

Effective supplements There is more good news. Several nutritional supplements have been found helpful against CHF, although they are not cures. One substance made by your body, known as coenzyme Q10, is often deficient in patients with heart failure according to the medical journal *Clinical Investigations* (vol. 71 (supplement), pp. 51–4, 1993). It also reported that heart failure patients with more coenzyme Q10 or vitamin E in their blood live longer.

Clinical trials, particularly in Italy, have now been carried out to see whether giving CHF patients 100 mg coenzyme Q10 per day could make a difference. The results have been reported in several medical journals: patients feel less tired, their ability to tolerate normal activity increases and they lose their breathing difficulties when resting.

Another nutritional supplement which has been found valuable in the treatment of CHF is the amino acid taurine. This nutrient regulates calcium and potassium in heart muscle cells, and in nerve impulses in the heart. Since magnesium is also involved in potassium balance, taurine is sometimes combined with magnesium and sold as a supplement known as magnesium taurate. (see Useful Addresses on p. 204 for suppliers).

CHAPTER

The Waterfall Diet

Now that you have identified some possible reasons why you might be retaining fluid, it is time for your treatment. The Waterfall Diet is *not* a low-calorie diet. It is about emphasizing some foods and avoiding others, not for reasons of their calorie content but to encourage the release of excess fluid. So it will not and should not leave you feeling hungry.

The diet is divided into three parts. Phase I, which you are recommended to follow for two months, is for all fluid retention sufferers. However, if you have been put on a special diet by a hospital dietician and told that it could be dangerous for you to deviate from it, ask your dietician's advice before considering the Waterfall Diet.

Phase I is designed to help clear your system of residues which may be encouraging fluid retention, and to provide the necessary raw materials for building up the strength of your blood capillaries and balancing your electrolytes, hormones and prostaglandins. Phase I is strict because this gets you the clearest and most rapid results. Although it does not restrict calories, Phase I does require you to abstain from foods which you may think of as staples, to shop for items which may seem unfamiliar, and to spend a little time in the kitchen preparing them.

Phase II, which takes four weeks, is similar to Phase I, but involves testing yourself for food allergies/intolerances which may have been contributing to your fluid retention. Again, whatever your type of fluid retention, you must complete Phase II. Your answers to the questionnaire in Chapter 2 will only offer a guide as to whether your fluid retention is likely to be caused by food allergy. Phases I and II of the Waterfall Diet will supply a much more definite answer.

Phase III is much more relaxed, and allows you a wide variety of foods. It is less a diet and more a long-term eating strategy, encouraging you to be conscious of foods that promote or fight your specific type of fluid retention and to eat accordingly. Occasional items are banned, but Phase III is mostly about encouraging a balance of 90 per cent beneficial foods, and 10 per cent free choice.

Phase I of the diet will result in rapid, almost immediate weight loss for allergic fluid retention, by taking away all the foods which might cause it. It is possible to lose up to 14 pounds in a week. For allergic people the remaining phases of the diet are concerned with identifying those foods so that in phase III you only need to avoid your own specific problem foods to keep the fluid retention away.

For other people following the diet, it will have a slower effect as the dietary changes promote the necessary repair work in the body to achieve good fluid balance. This is why two months is advised for Phase I. Allergic people too need this repair work since the avoidance of problem foods is only a palliative measure (like taking a diuretic medicine).

Phase III is for keeping the fluid retention away; that is why it is described as a permanent eating strategy.

Phase I

Phase I of the Waterfall Diet involves three vital principles:

- Avoiding even small amounts of the 'Not Allowed' foods (see table opposite)
- Consuming the beneficial foods as frequently as possible (see table on p. 137).
- Balancing foods to ensure the greatest possible variety. For example, you will not succeed on this diet if you avoid all vegetables. You must find some way to consume them, even if you make them into soups and juices.

Provided that you stick with these three principles, you will be

Food and Ingredients not Allowed in Phase I of the Waterfall Diet

More information about the suggested alternatives is given on pp. 156–162.

Food	Reason
Coffee	Diuretic effect. Can make high-protein type fluid retention worse: diuretics encourage dehydration and so make your kidneys retain sodium (and therefore water) because the excess protein in your tissue spaces must be kept diluted. Coffee also causes loss of magnesium and other minerals and increases your liver's workload. ALTERNATIVES: Chicory and dandelion coffee
Sugar, honey, syrup, and foods containing added sugar. Read your labels, since sugar is also known as sucrose, glucose, dextrose and fructose.	Sugar is absorbed into your blood and turned into glucose much more quickly than any other foods. This can make your insulin levels rise too fast and too much. These excess insulin levels make you retain sodium (and therefore water) and encourage fatty deposits in arteries and as stored body fat, especially around your middle! 　　Large amounts of sugar also seem to have a harmful effect on the kidneys and can cause them to become enlarged (see p. 33). 　　Excess sugar encourages deficiencies of vitamins, minerals and flavonoids needed for strong blood capillary walls, since it is very high in calories yet contains no nutrients of its own. This has the effect of diluting more nutrient-rich foods like lean meat and vegetables. ALTERNATIVES: Use naturally sweet foods like bananas, raisins, dates and carob.
1. Salt, and highly salted or smoked foods such as salami, ham and bacon, smoked fish, salty cheeses, stock cubes, yeast extract, soy sauce and bought pies, quiches sauces and 'oven-ready' dishes. 2. Sodium-rich drinks, medicines and food additives. Baking powder. Most commercial soft drinks are very high in	There is a direct relationship between the amount of salt or sodium you consume and the amount of fluid you retain. Reducing your salt or sodium consumption will immediately result in some loss of retained fluid since water always follows sodium. ALTERNATIVES: Potassium salt, miso, potassium baking powder. To make the diet more palatable a small amount of tamari sauce (wheat-free soy sauce) is included in some of the recipes.

Food	Reason

sodium. Some medicines, such as antacids based on bicarbonate of soda, and effervescent tablets, can also contain much sodium. A common food additive is the flavour-enhancer monosodium glutamate or 'E621'. Other sodium-rich food additives are E211, E223, E250, E251, E262(ii), E281, E339, E350, E401, E452, E466, E500, E514, E524, R541, E576.

Fat, and especially saturated fat, in large amounts as found in fatty minced beef and burgers, sausages, pork pies, chocolate, crisps, fried food, butter, margarine, cream, cheese, mayonnaise, pastry, and many sauces, dips and desserts.

Fat is not a poison; in fact it is essential to have some fat (in the form of essential polyunsaturated oils) in your diet. But many of us consume too much of the foods listed opposite, which can contain invisible fat. A high-fat diet can encourage fluid retention in several ways:
• In time it may impair kidney function.
• It will also encourage deficiencies of vitamins, minerals and flavonoids needed for strong blood capillary walls, since it is very high in calories yet contains few nutrients of its own. As with sugar, this has the effect of diluting more nutrient-rich foods like lean meat and vegetables.
• Animal fat contains arachidonic acid, which can encourage inflammation in your skin, joints or other parts of your body, and therefore fluid retention.
ALTERNATIVES TO SATURATED FAT: Oils, especially extra virgin olive oil and unrefined sunflower or soya oil. Also nuts and seeds used in meals will provide the essential polyunsaturated oils that your body needs and will help to make a meal filling.

White flour

White flour is often more enjoyable than wholemeal in foods like cakes, biscuits, sauces, pastry and pasta. Some people also prefer it in bread. But white flour is almost devoid of important minerals like magnesium and zinc, and is so poor in B vitamins that by law some have to be artificially replaced! Once you have reduced your fluid retention, eat foods made from white flour if your type of fluid retention permits it, but remember that the more of them you eat, the more you risk inadequately nourishing your body.

White flour is also a very poor source of dietary fibre, which is needed to prevent constipation. See p. 77 for some of the important reasons for avoiding constipation.

ALTERNATIVES: Brown rice flour is light in colour and texture and can be used in baking if recipes are adapted to take into account its lack of gluten. Some health shops are now selling the 'Stamp Collection All Purpose' flour (and similar products) which can be used in white flour recipes and is made from barley, rice, millet and maize.

Alcohol	Alcohol stresses your liver and reduces the effectiveness of anti-diuretic hormone (ADH), a hormone which slows down your kidneys' excretion of fluid when your body's fluid levels are getting low. So alcohol can cause dehydration by encouraging rapid water excretion even when body fluid levels are already low. As mentioned above, dehydration is especially undesirable if you suffer from high-protein type fluid retention. ALTERNATIVES: See the suggested drinks on p. 195.
Artificial food additives	It is hard to avoid these if you eat commercially manufactured foods. Almost everything contains a cocktail of additives: preservatives, colourings, artificial sweeteners, flavourings and flavour enhancers to name just a few. Sometimes the law does not even require additives to be listed on a packet. For instance a chilled meal purchased from a supermarket may appear to contain no additives at all, but this is because items like stock do not have to declare small amounts of sub-ingredients which they contain.

The problem with additives is that we only know if they harm the health of well-nourished laboratory animals given them singly in large quantities. We have no idea how they affect the health of humans when consumed over a lifetime in dozens of different combinations.

Some additives are known to trigger problems like asthma and skin rashes in children. Others have been banned after it was discovered that they were unsafe. |

Food	Reason
	Your liver must try to break down these foreign chemicals, and uses up its precious resources in doing so. ALTERNATIVES: There are now many additive-free products on the market. Health food shops often specialize in them. Or make your own additive-free food.
Potential allergens: wheat (and bread, pasta etc. made from wheat), dairy produce, eggs and yeast	Almost all people who suffer from the kind of food intolerances which lead to fluid retention (see Chapter 2) will improve if they avoid these four foods. So Phase I of the Waterfall Diet excludes these foods to help you release any fluid which they may have been causing. You can test them one by one in Phase II to see if any particular one brings a return of your fluid retention. ALTERNATIVES TO WHEAT: Spelt, rice, barley, rye, millet flour etc. ALTERNATIVES TO MILK: Soya milk, nut milk, rice milk. ALTERNATIVES TO EGGS: In cakes, a mixture of soya flour and soya milk can often replace eggs due to the high protein content. ALTERNATIVES TO BREAD MADE WITH YEAST: Yeast- and wheat-free rye bread. Or make your own spelt flour griddle bread or oat pancakes (see pp. 194 and 188). ALTERNATIVES TO STOCK CUBES AND GRAVY MIXES CONTAINING YEAST: Miso.
Red meat of all types and non-organically farmed white meat	Red meat (even if apparently lean) and saturated fat contain arachidonic acid, which can encourage inflammation in your skin, joints or other parts of your body, and therefore fluid retention. White meat (poultry) is much less fatty, but avoid it during Phase I unless it has been organically raised. Even free-range chickens may be fed standard commercial feed which contains antibiotics, dung from other chickens, and other unsavoury items. We do not know how well a chicken's liver can cope with these challenges and what kind of residues remain in the bird's meat and fat. ALTERNATIVES: Fish, tofu and other soya products.

Note: If it seems like all your favourite foods are forbidden, don't worry. Phase I of the Waterfall Diet only lasts for two months and its benefits start very quickly. Meanwhile, there are lots of delicious alternatives, and while you are spending the first few weeks trying them out you will gradually miss your old favourites less and less.

Foods at a Glance: Good or Bad for Fluid Retention?

Count up the number of ticks for a particular food; the more ticks it has, the better it works against fluid retention

Food	Not a Common Allergen*	Protein Rich	Low in Potentially Harmful Fat Content	Low in Sodium	Low in Added Sugar	Helps Your Liver	Good Source of Vitamin B6	Rich in Magnesium	Rich in Many Vitamins and Minerals	Rich in Essential Polyunsaturated Oils	Low in Arachidonic Acid	Rich in Flavonoids	Rich in Coumarin	Rich in Dietary Fibre
Apples	✓	✓	✓	✓	✓						✓	✓		✓
Avocados	✓	✓	✓	✓	✓		✓	✓	✓	✓	✓	✓		✓
X Bacon (lean)	✓	✓	✓		✓		✓		✓					
Bananas	✓		✓	✓	✓		✓	✓	✓		✓			✓
X Butter					✓									
Beans	✓	✓	✓	✓	✓		✓	✓	✓		✓	✓		✓
X Beer			✓	✓	✓		✓				✓	✓		

Continued

Food	Not a Common Allergen*	Protein Rich	Low in Potentially Harmful Fat Content	Low in Sodium	Low in Added Sugar	Helps Your Liver	Good Source of Vitamin B6	Rich in Magnesium	Rich in Many Vitamins and Minerals	Rich in Essential Polyunsaturated Oils	Low in Arachidonic Acid	Rich in Flavonoids	Rich in Coumarin	Rich in Dietary Fibre
Beetroot,	✓		✓	✓	✓	✓			✓		✓			✓
Bilberries blueberries, blackberries, black grapes and black cherries	✓		✓	✓	✓	✓			✓		✓	✓		✓
✗< Bitter chocolate	✓	✓	✓	✓				✓	✓		✓			
✗ Bread (commercial, white)		✓	✓	✓	✓						✓			

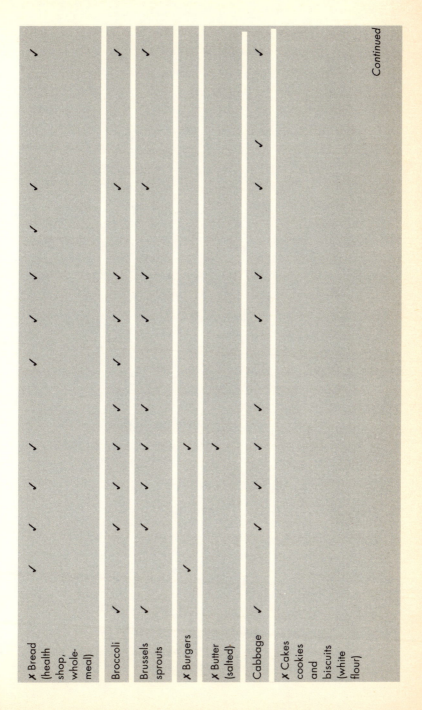

x Bread (health shop, wholemeal)

Broccoli

Brussels sprouts

x Burgers

x Butter (salted)

Cabbage

x Cakes cookies and biscuits (white flour)

Continued

Food	Not a Common Allergen*	Protein Rich	Low in Potentially Harmful Fat Content	Low in Sodium	Low in Added Sugar	Helps Your Liver	Good Source of Vitamin B6	Rich in Magnesium	Rich in Many Vitamins and Minerals	Rich in Essential Polyunsaturated Oils	Low in Arachidonic Acid	Rich in Flavonoids	Rich in Coumarin	Rich in Dietary Fibre
Carrots	✓		✓	✓	✓				✓		✓			✓
Cauliflower	✓		✓	✓	✓	✓			✓		✓			✓
Celery	✓		✓	✓	✓				✓		✓	✓	✓	✓
✗ Cheese		✓		✓	✓				✓					
Cherries (Black)	✓		✓	✓	✓				✓		✓	✓		✓
✗ Colas and similar artificial drinks			✓								✓			
✗ Coffee	✓		✓	✓	✓									

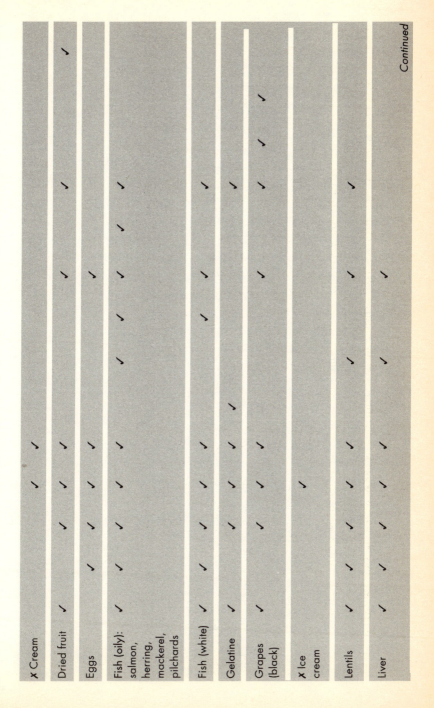

x Cream

Dried fruit

Eggs

Fish (oily): salmon, herring, mackerel, pilchards

Fish (white)

Gelatine

Grapes (black)

x Ice cream

Lentils

Liver

Continued

Food	Not a Common Allergen*	Protein Rich	Low in Potentially Harmful Fat Content	Low in Sodium	Low in Added Sugar	Helps Your Liver	Good Source of Vitamin B6	Rich in Magnesium	Rich in Many Vitamins and Minerals	Rich in Essential Polyunsaturated Oils	Low in Arachidonic Acid	Rich in Flavonoids	Rich in Coumarin	Rich in Dietary Fibre
x Margarine					✓					✓				
x Meat (red)	✓	✓		✓	✓		✓							
☺ Meat (white)	✓	✓	✓	✓	✓		✓		✓					
x Milk (cow's, full fat)		✓		✓	✓				✓					
Milk (sheep or goat's)	✓	✓		✓	✓				✓					
x Milk chocolate		✓		✓										
Nuts and seeds	✓	✓	✓	✓	✓		✓	✓	✓		✓			

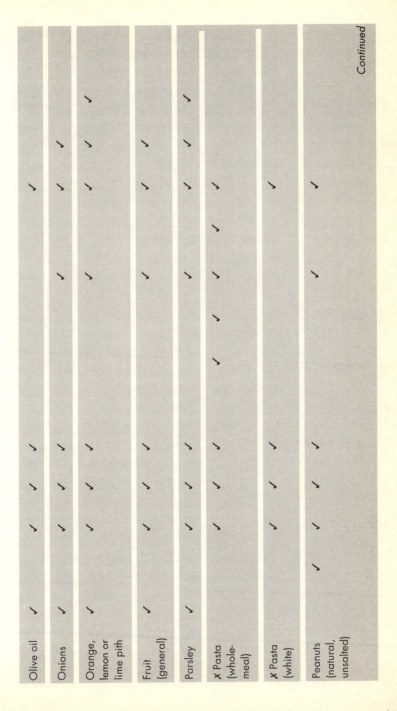

- Olive oil
- Onions
- Orange, lemon or lime pith
- Fruit (general)
- Parsley
- x Pasta (wholemeal)
- x Pasta (white)
- Peanuts (natural, unsalted)

Continued

Food	Not a Common Allergen*	Protein Rich	Low in Potentially Harmful Fat Content	Low in Sodium	Low in Added Sugar	Helps Your Liver	Good Source of Vitamin B6	Rich in Magnesium	Rich in Many Vitamins and Minerals	Rich in Essential Polyunsatured Oils	Low in Arachidonic Acid	Rich in Flavonoids	Rich in Coumarin	Rich in Dietary Fibre
Peppers and horse-radish	✓		✓	✓	✓				✓		✓		✓	
Porridge oats	✓		✓	✓	✓			✓	✓	✓	✓			
Potatoes	✓		✓	✓	✓		✓	✓	✓					
Rice (brown)	✓		✓	✓	✓		✓	✓	✓	✓	✓			
x Rice (white)	✓		✓	✓	✓				✓		✓			
Soya flour	✓	✓	✓	✓	✓			✓	✓	✓	✓			
Soya milk	✓	✓	✓	✓	✓			✓	✓	✓	✓			

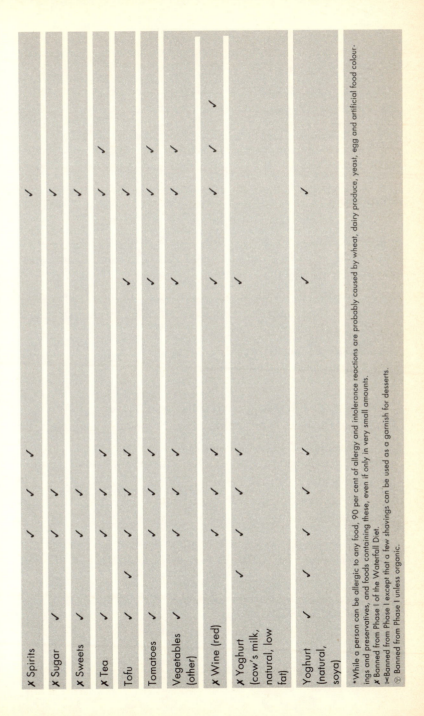

*While a person can be allergic to any food, 90 per cent of allergy and intolerance reactions are probably caused by wheat, dairy produce, yeast, egg and artificial food colourings and preservatives, and foods containing these, even if only in very small amounts.

x Banned from Phase I of the Waterfall Diet.

✗ Banned from Phase I except that a few shavings can be used as a garnish for desserts.

Ⓢ Banned from Phase I unless organic.

able to construct your own menus. To help you get started, I have included some suggestions for meals and some recipes, which are almost all quick and easy. A Waterfall Diet Cookbook is also in preparation. Try to vary your choices as much as possible rather than, for instance, eating the same breakfast every day. Any of the meal suggestions given can be used at any time of day. For information on where to find the ingredients and how to prepare them, see p. 156.

Breakfast

This is the most important meal of the day, especially if you are slimming. When you sleep your body is fasting and its metabolism slows down. Eating a good breakfast stimulates your metabolism to speed up again, thus burning off your calories faster. Missing breakfast means keeping your metabolism slow until lunch time, and will also leave you lacking in energy and feeling comparatively stressed and irritable.

Some people avoid breakfast because it leaves them feeling hungry again very soon afterwards. This only happens when your breakfast consists mainly of carbohydrate, which sends your blood sugar up and then quickly down again, resulting in hunger. The breakfast ideas given below should not have this effect, as they contain protein and essential polyunsaturated oils.

Any of the following are suitable for this diet, but oats are a particularly good breakfast food because they are rich in magnesium, B vitamins, essential polyunsaturated oils and soluble fibre. This helps to keep your blood sugar on an even keel and prevent early hunger.

- Sheep's milk or soya yoghurt with apple compote and almonds (see p. 170)
- Sultana and sunflower seed porridge with soya milk and soya cream (see p. 170)
- Authentic Swiss muesli with flaked nuts and sweet apricots (see p. 170)
- Warm Derbyshire oatcakes (see p. 188) with sugar-free black cherry jam and crunchy nut butter.

- Cornflakes with sliced bananas, cashew nuts and soya milk
- Brown rice pudding (see p. 186) with crushed brazil nuts and sugar-free marmalade
- Avocado 'smoothie' with soya milk, banana and strawberries (see p. 171)

Lunch

If you work at home, you can use any of the recipes in this book for lunch. Otherwise you will need to make yourself a packed lunch. Do make sure you are always prepared. Essential stand-bys which ensure that you will always be able to whip up a packed lunch without much forethought are:

- Cooked brown rice
- Cooked beans
- Miso
- Red and green peppers
- Left-over steamed vegetable pieces such as carrots or broccoli
- Tinned sardines in olive oil or tomato
- Fresh parsley
- Soya yoghurt
- Raw white cabbage

The rice, beans and vegetables or chopped peppers can be combined with some French dressing and chopped parsley to make a salad, served with tinned sardines. The raw cabbage can be finely shredded and combined with soya yoghurt and a few drops of cider vinegar or lemon juice to make coleslaw. Add boiling water to a teaspoon of miso for a nutritious instant soup.

Another good standby is a large pan of chunky fresh vegetable soup kept in the fridge. Buy a wide-neck thermos flask, heat up the soup in the morning and take it in the thermos to work. Dunk it with oatcakes or griddle bread (see pp. 188 and 194), or stuff a griddle bread with hummus (see p. 189) and salad.

Protein-rich bean salad can be made from your stock of frozen beans prepared as described on p. 158. Just defrost a mixture of kidney beans, chick peas and white haricot beans overnight, and combine with French dressing (see p. 191) and chopped parsley in the morning.

If you run out of ideas, here are a few to keep you going:

- Shredded white cabbage with grated carrot in soya yoghurt and mustard vinaigrette (see p. 173)
- Broccoli in vinaigrette with sliced spring onion (see p. 174)
- Avocado with French dressing (see p. 191) and black pepper.
- Tomato slices on a bed of alfalfa and grated radish sprinkled with French dressing (see p. 174) and topped with tofu mayonnaise (see p. 191)
- Yeast- and wheat-free pumpernickel bread or Ryvita

Plus
- Cream of Brussels sprout, broccoli, celery or cauliflower soup (see p. 172)
- Chunky winter vegetable soup with marrowfat peas (see p. 172)
- Lentil soup with miso, celery and onion (see p. 173)

Plus
- 1 portion cold roast organic chicken *or* tofu kebab *or* bean and vegetable rosti *or* portion of unsalted canned pilchards/sardines

Plus
- 1 apple *or* orange (including some of the white pith) *or* black cherries *or* grapes *or* blueberries

For suggestions for main meals, desserts and snacks see the Recipe section.

Drinks

If you normally drink only tea and coffee, you may have come to believe that all your drinks should be brown! Naturally this is not true. There are hundreds of good drinks waiting to be tried, though you may find it hard at first to break old habits.

All the following drinks are suitable for the Waterfall Diet. The home-made juices are concentrated plant nutrition in a glass, so they also have a highly therapeutic effect. You should try to drink at least one large glass a day of them. But don't stick to one – you will gain more benefit if you rotate them.

You will have to look in a health food shop to find some of the other suggested drinks.

Therapeutic drinks
- Home-made apple, celery, parsley and radish juice (see p. 196)
- Beetroot juice (either home-made or from shop), mixed with celery and lemon juice (see p. 196)
- Home-made broccoli stem and sharp apple juice (see p. 196)
- Home-made flavonoid-rich orange juice (see p. 197); make with a juice extractor rather than with a citrus juicer, and leave some of the white pith on the fruit
- Herbal teas: fennel, comfrey, chamomile, nettle, parsley
- Home-made clover tea: pick clover blossoms, dry them (see p. 197) to bring out the coumarin
- Plain water (preferably filtered or bottled)

Other Drinks
- Fresh orange juice mixed with sparking mineral water
- Iced herbal or rose-hip tea
- Chicory or dandelion coffee with soya milk
- Green tea (no more than two cups a week, as this is high in caffeine)
- Decaffeinated black tea with soya or sheep's milk
- Home-made fresh ginger tea with lemon zest

(Do not add sugar, honey, sweeteners or cow's milk to any of these drinks)

Snack ideas (see also Recipes)
- Fruit, especially black grapes, berries, apples and oranges
- Celery sticks and raw carrot sticks
- Handful of brazil nuts/sunflower seeds/almonds/cashew nuts
- Unsalted dry roast peanuts
- Oatcakes with nut butter and sugar-free jam
- Any leftover dessert or breakfast items, or items from main meals which can be eaten cold
- Bowl of hot vegetable soup with oatcakes

Useful Hints And Tips For Getting Through Phase I

Getting started Don't start the Waterfall Diet until you are properly organized. If you shop weekly in a supermarket, check that it can provide everything you need. If not, ask in your local health food shop. If trying to save money, buy your fish and vegetables from a fishmonger and greengrocer – they will be cheaper. Check the availability of organic chicken and vegetables from your local organic supplier, or see Useful Addresses on p. 202 for national suppliers.

Check that the diet will work into your schedule. If you usually come home hungry after working late, and grab something quick from the fridge, you will need to make sure that it's going to be compatible with this diet.

Make lots of thick bean and vegetable stews to keep in the fridge to heat up quickly when you get home – or put them in a 'slow cooker' so that delicious smells will waft through the door to greet you. Cook a large pan of brown rice and when cold freeze it in portions ready for defrosting and quickly heating up when

needed. Do the same with a packet of dried peas or beans. Since you will probably need packed lunches if you go out to work, organize these the night before.

Proper preparations will make the Waterfall Diet much easier and more enjoyable. The first week is the most difficult time; if you can get through that you will probably succeed and reap all the benefits which the diet brings. You may lose not only your fluid retention but a host of minor problems such as sleeping difficulties, occasional headaches, spotty skin, constipation, bloating, sore joints, premenstrual symptoms and lack of energy.

Equipment Although not vital, you will find it much easier to follow the Waterfall Diet if you have access to a freezer and a pressure cooker; the latter is especially good for dried pulses, because it can cook them in a few minutes whereas ordinary boiling can take hours. Do also try to get a juice extractor, since otherwise you will not be able to extract the concentrated nutrients from celery, radishes and other fruit and vegetables which can help to combat your fluid retention.

'I haven't got time to cook!'

Everyone has time to cook, but not everyone makes cooking a priority! Most of us have also got out of the habit of regular cooking because it is so much easier to buy ready-made foods.

With the Waterfall Diet, an hour or two spent in the kitchen can result in mountains of food ready for freezing or storing in the fridge for instant use over the next few days. For instance a large pan of soup will last four or five days, a bag of frozen brown rice (see p. 195) will give you up to half a dozen meals, and a bag of frozen beans (see p. 195) will provide masses of great-value instant protein.

Just stir-fry these two ingredients with some olive oil, herbs, pepper and potassium salt, add cooked fresh vegetables, and you will have a meal far cheaper and just as quick as anything you can buy ready-made, but with far more health benefits. Or pop some frozen butter beans into a large pan of cooked, liquidized carrots, potatoes, leeks and onions, heat through and add soya cream. What could be simpler?

A frozen fillet of sole takes minutes to defrost in hot water and then grill. You can also make liberal use of frozen vegetables and leftover fresh vegetables. In fact why not make a point of cooking more vegetables than you need so that you have enough to last you for a few days, heated up with steamed potato pieces in a tightly lidded pan with some olive oil and a few tablespoons of water. Serve with your grilled fish.

Check labels carefully Most commercial foods have a habit of including small amounts of wheat, egg, yeast or dairy produce in the small print, so do make sure you study labels on packets before buying, and if you don't know what terms like 'modified starch' or 'casein' mean, assume that to be on the safe side you can't have them. Home-made is best, since you know exactly what you have put into each dish.

Getting enough calcium

Since Phase I of the Waterfall Diet allows no cow's milk or dairy produce, your friends and family could become concerned that you might not get enough calcium, particularly if you are worried about preventing brittle bone disease (osteoporosis). Some doctors and dieticians, too, may try to pressurize you into consuming milk and cheese because these are the easiest ways to obtain this essential mineral. If in doubt, contact the Vegan Society (see Useful Addresses on p. 202), which can provide scientific information written by qualified state-registered dieticians on the health and safety of dairy-free diets.

Almonds and carob flour are a particularly rich source of calcium, followed by dark green leafy vegetables like kale and broccoli, and sunflower or sesame seeds, brazil nuts and tofu.

Getting enough protein As you know, a protein deficiency can encourage fluid retention, so it is important to eat enough protein every day. The meal plans suggested for the Waterfall Diet take this into account, but if you try to adapt them, remember that you must consume a good portion of at least one of the following foods at each meal: nuts or seeds (e.g. sunflower seeds), pulses (e.g. beans, lentils, tofu or soya flour), brown rice, fish or organic chicken. Don't get stuck on just one or two of these for convenience's sake; most plant proteins are not complete proteins and as much variety as possible should be consumed.

Coping with sugar cravings
Such cravings can be hard to cope with, especially if you are not allowed artificial sweeteners either. Sugary foods tend to be our 'comfort' foods. In avoiding them we feel we are being deprived of comfort as well as enjoyment.

So you will be very pleased to know that the most harmful effect of sugar consumption – its tendency to raise insulin levels too quickly and too high – can be largely prevented if you eat naturally sweet foods rather than foods with added sugar. This is because the natural sugars in these foods are bound tightly to the dietary fibre they contain, and the digestive process cannot separate the two very quickly. This results in a slower absorption of sugar, and a more gradual rise in insulin levels.

Naturally sweet foods include apples, oranges, bananas, sultanas, dates, dried apricots and other dried fruit, but honey and natural syrups are not permitted since these have a similar effect on your metabolism to ordinary sugar.

If you sweeten your snacks and desserts with naturally sweet foods, you will hardly notice that you are unable to eat sugar.

Coping with chocolate cravings While it is an acquired taste, a craving for chocolate may have started with an attempt by your body to get more of the minerals magnesium and iron, which are found in cocoa powder. Since the Waterfall Diet provides healthy amounts of both minerals, it should help you to lose any physical addiction to chocolate. This just leaves the psychological cravings of comfort eating!

The best way to deal with this is to eat or drink something else which makes you feel that you have had a treat. Alternatively, make yourself a delicious choco-late banana cream boat using the recipe on p. 184. Using only a little cocoa powder, it will give you the taste of chocolate without the excess fat and sugar, and will help with that element of comfort.

And after all, treats don't have to be edible – you could buy yourself something new to wear, or have a new hairdo, or do something special that you have been promising yourself for years but never got around to: learning to ride a horse or a motorbike, planning a Caribbean cruise or taking up a creative new hobby. You may soon have a brand-new figure to do it in!

Coping with business lunches, restaurants and dining out Many business exec-utives feel very pressured to be one of the lads when it comes to wining and dining. But the truth is that most of the business world is becoming increasingly health-conscious, and you may well find that your client or host is also on a diet. Brazen it out, and explain that your diet is just temporary. Tell them about it. They may even want to join you in adopting it!

Opting for mineral water, grilled fish or roast chicken and vegeta-bles, followed by fruit, is usually possible in most restaurants. Ethnic restaurants often offer plain rice and vegetable or lentil dishes, rice noodles, tofu, fish and other non-meat options, though beware monosodium glutamate in Chinese thickened sauces, and a possibly excessive use of soy sauce, which is high in salt. Japanese sushi is often compatible with Phase I of the Waterfall Diet.

As far as dining out is concerned, do tell your friends that you are on a diet, and let anyone who is going to cook for you have a list of permitted ingredients. They may well be very interested and keen to accommodate you. Perhaps they too will want to take up the diet themselves!

I am sometimes asked, 'What can I do if, due to completely unforeseen circumstances, there is absolutely nothing suitable for me to eat?' Some of the least harmful occasional sins during Phase I of this diet would include ordinary fried or roast chicken (no coating), chips, white rice (but not white bread or other wheat-containing food), fried fish with the batter removed, and 'special fried rice' containing small pieces

of chicken, pork etc.

What can I have to drink?

Tea, coffee, cola and beer are not essentials – water is! Drinking water in preference to other drinks helps to dilute the fluid in your tissue spaces; as explained on p. 86, the more dilute it is, the more easily it can get back into your blood capillaries. While tap water contains a lot of chlorine and other impurities, bottled water can work out quite expensive, so you may want to invest in a water filter.

Using tinned and frozen foods

These foods can be great time-savers, but must comply with the general rules of the Waterfall Diet. So in Phase I, where products containing sugar are not allowed, you would not be able to eat fruit preserved in syrup (which is made from sugar), but plain frozen fruit or fruit canned or bottled in its own juice is the next best thing to fresh. Likewise frozen vegetables or Italian plum tomatoes canned in their own juice are all right, but try to avoid brands containing artificial additives. Other types of canned vegetables are probably high in salt and should be avoided. Do remember that, while convenience is sometimes important, fresh is always best for your body, because the longer food is stored, the more nutrients like vitamin C and some of the B vitamins are destroyed.

Coping with side effects from the Waterfall Diet Most people are likely to experience side-effects from the Waterfall Diet – usually caffeine withdrawal symptoms in the form of a nagging headache for a day or two. Take plain soluble aspirin if it becomes difficult to cope with, but do not take paracetamol (acetaminophen) or other painkillers since these are usually more stressful to your liver.

Other potential side-effects are weakness and fatigue if you do not eat enough calories. Don't try to kill two birds with one stone by also turning this into a very low-calorie diet – you will not gain the maximum benefit from it if you do. Instead of concentrating on the long-term adjustments to your eating habits that you must make after Phases I and II to keep your fluid retention away, you will be desperate to come off this diet and

resume eating all the foods that were giving you fluid retention.

Remember that to keep up your calorie intake, you will probably need to eat *more* food than usual on the Waterfall Diet – especially for breakfast and lunch. Although you may have been used to no more than a cup of coffee and a sandwich, with a couple of bars of chocolate in between, the calories in a bar of chocolate can be the equivalent of a whole meal on the Waterfall Diet!

If you are not used to eating a fibre-rich diet like the Waterfall Diet, you may react with more wind or looser bowel motions than usual. It will settle down eventually; just eat little and often for the time being, and avoid eating large amounts of any particularly problematic foods.

What if I just can't get to grips with the diet and want to give up? The recommended time to spend on Phase I is two months. This gives your body time to carry out quite a lot of repair work on the damage caused by any previous faulty eating habits or by special nutritional needs going unfulfilled. But if you feel that you can't cope with two months, set yourself a target of two weeks instead. If you want to give up after two weeks and move on to Phase II, you can, and you will still have received a lot of benefits. On the other hand, most people find that after managing it for two weeks they have got over most of the problems and the rest is plain sailing. You might even find that it takes a couple of practice runs to get into it, so don't lose heart. If you can't manage the full two months the first time, you might be able to next year, for instance.

Using Unfamiliar Ingredients

Ingredient	Where to Get It	What It's Good for	How to Use It
Alfalfa sprouts	Health food shops (seeds also sold)	Rich in coumarin	Alfalfa sprouts can be bought in packets, but it is cheaper to make your own. Place a level tablespoon of seeds in a large jar, then cover the jar with a piece of nylon fabric from an old pair of tights and secure the fabric with an elastic band around the neck of the jar. Run some water into the jar, shake to wet the seeds thoroughly, then leave overnight. In the morning, pour the water away, straining it through the nylon cover. Rinse the seeds by pouring in water and immediately straining it out again morning and night, and in a few days you will have a luscious growth of curly green sprouts which can be added to soups or eaten as salad. Eat them when they are about 1 inch long. You can also follow the same procedure to sprout lentils, mung beans, aduki beans, black buckwheat grains, barley grains, almonds and clover seeds.

continued

Ingredient	Where to Get It	What It's Good for	How to Use It
Bilberries	Frozen food departments of some larger supermarkets	Rich in flavonoids	Allow to defrost, then consume them as they are, or place in an oven-proof casserole dish in a medium oven for 25 minutes or until the fruits split and the juices run. Serve hot or cold, with soya cream, or combine with gelatine or vegetarian gelling product before cooling to make bilberry jelly. If sweetening is required, use a small amount of puréed dates (see p. 192).
Blue-berries	Fruit departments of some larger supermarkets or superstores. Some health shops may also sell sugar-free blueberry jam.	Rich in flavonoids	Serve fresh with soya yoghurt, or cook as for bilberries. Should need no sweetening as blueberries are sweeter than bilberries. Use blueberry jam as any other jam.
Brown rice	Supermarkets and health food shops	Rich in B vitamins	Brown rice is nuttier than white rice and has a different texture. Wash thoroughly, then pre-soak overnight in twice its volume of filtered water. Use the same water for cooking. Bring to the boil, then cover tightly and simmer on the lowest possible heat for 20 minutes. If the water has not all been absorbed, drain away the excess (or save it for adding to soup, as it is very rich in vitamins), then leave the rice in the covered saucepan away from the heat for 5 minutes, after which it is ready to serve. Once cold, brown rice can be spread out on an oiled baking tray, frozen, then crumbled into grains and bagged for the freezer.

Buck-wheat	Health food shops	Rich in magnesium and in the flavonoid rutin, which helps to build capillary strength	Buckwheat is a grain unrelated to wheat and is a good alternative for wheat allergy sufferers. The grains can be cooked like rice, or are available as a flour which contains no gluten and is the main ingredient of the small Russian pancakes known as blinis. To cook buckwheat grains, soak overnight in twice their volume of water, then bring to the boil and simmer very gently with the lid on for 15–20 minutes, or until the grains are tender. Use as an alternative to rice.
Carob flour	Health food shops	Very rich in calcium. Naturally sweet and often used as a healthier alternative to cocoa	The carob is a type of bean. It is made into flour which can be incorporated in cakes and biscuits to give a light brown colour and natural sweetness.
Dandelion coffee	Health food shops	Helps to drain the liver and gall bladder	Can be bought as granules and used as instant coffee. If you find it lacks flavour, try mixing it with chicory coffee.
Dried beans, split peas, chickpeas, marrow-fat peas	Supermarkets, grocers and health food shops	A very cheap source of protein, rich in dietary fibre	These should be soaked in water before use. Cover with four times their volume in boiling filtered water and leave overnight. Throw away the soaking water, then place the beans, just covered with fresh water, in a pressure cooker, bring to full steam, and cook for 3–8 minutes, depending on size. Pressure-cooking breaks down the poisonous lectins found in raw beans. If

continued

Ingredient	Where to Get It	What It's Good for	How to Use It
			you do not have a pressure cooker, boil them fast for at least 10 minutes before simmering or slow-cooking. Conventional boiling can take 2 hours or more to soften them, depending on age and size. To freeze, allow to cool and follow the same procedure as for frozen brown rice.
Herbal teas	Health food shops	Often rich in flavonoids, coumarin or other beneficial ingredients.	Some beneficial teas are buckwheat, chamomile, clover blossom, nettle, parsley and comfrey teas, or a mixture of any of these. Comfrey has had a very unjust bad press. In a government report which claimed that comfrey causes liver damage to animals, most of the cases reported were in fact caused by other plants containing similar but much more poisonous alkaloids. A man in Australia was reported to have died from eating fresh comfrey leaves when comfrey was not even in season. In a 1993 survey carried out in the UK on 600 comfrey users, not one person reported experiencing any of the health problems that are claimed to result from it. Only benefits were experienced, including considerable relief from arthritis and digestive problems. A copy of this report is available free of charge to medical or research institutions, from the Society for the Promotion of Nutritional Therapy (see Useful Addresses, on p. 202).

Lentils (red, green, brown, puy and other varieties)	Lentils are widely available, but health food shops tend to provide the widest choice	Rich in protein and dietary fibre or soup. No pre-soaking required.	Use to make lentil curry (dahl) Lentils take 20–30 minutes to cook, depending on size.
Miso	Health food shops	Dark brown stock paste. Unlike most stock paste, miso is very rich in vitamins and minerals and lower in sodium. It also contains protein	Mix with boiling water and use to make gravy and to flavour dark soups and stews. One variety of miso is made with wheat, and should be avoided during Phases I and II of the Waterfall Diet. Other types, such as barley miso, are all right. Don't overdo the miso – it does contain salt. Use just enough to get some colour and flavour into a dish.
Oats	Widely available. Health food shops sell organically grown oats	Rich in B vitamins, magnesium and dietary fibre	Make rolled oats into porridge for breakfast, or soak oatmeal in water overnight to make a creamy muesli. Oats are also used to make flapjacks and oat biscuits.
Potassium baking powder	Health food shops	Allows you to bake cakes, scones and biscuits without the added sodium found in ordinary baking powder	Use in accordance with the manufacturer's directions on the container.
Potassium salt (Ruthmol)	Health food shops	Allows you to season your food without sodium, and increases valuable potassium	Add to food as you would ordinary salt. Potassium salt is also found in 'low salt' products which consist of half to two-thirds potassium salt and the rest ordinary sodium salt.

continued

Ingredient	Where to Get It	What It's Good for	How to Use It
Pumpernickel bread	Supermarkets, health food shops	Wholegrain rye bread with a sweetish, nutty flavour. Buy a brand which contains no yeast or wheat	Eat with soups and salads, or make into an open sandwich (to eat with a knife and fork) by spreading with hummus and adding salad toppings. Pumpernickel does contain a very small amount of salt, but this should not be a problem.
Sheep's milk yoghurt	Supermarkets	An alternative to cow's milk yoghurt	Use as normal yoghurt.
Soya cream	Health food shops	A blend of soya protein and oil which can be used as an alternative to dairy single cream	Soya cream is used as a topping for desserts, or can be stirred into soup or gravy to achieve the same effect as single cream. Look for it under brand names such as Provamel's 'Soya Dream'.
Soya flour	Health food shops	High in protein. Provides all the benefits of soy foods, including protection against prostate cancer and menopausal problems	A few tablespoons of soya flour can often be used as an alternative to eggs in baking because of its high protein content.
Soya milk	Widely available	Provides all the benefits of soy foods	Use in the same way as cow's milk. Contains less protein, calcium and fat, but a good balance of vitamins and minerals. Some brands are enriched with calcium. Cook slowly with brown rice to make great rice pudding.

Soya yoghurt	Health food shops. If you have difficulty finding it, ask for plain Yofu or Sojasun, which is a good thick brand. Or make your own.	An alternative to cow's milk yoghurt. Provides all the benefits of soy foods, plus the friendly bacteria found in normal yoghurt.	Use as normal yoghurt.
Spelt flour	Health food shops	An alternative to wholewheat flour. Most people who are allergic to wheat are not allergic to spelt.	Use exactly as wholewheat flour. You can also buy pasta made from spelt.
Sugar-free black cherry jam	Some larger supermarkets and superstores sell the excellent St Dalfour brand	Black cherry skins are rich in flavonoids, and so is the grape juice used to sweeten this jam	Use as normal jam.
Sugar-free marma-lade	Health food shops. Also St Dalfour Thick Cut Orange Spread	Citrus peel is rich in flavonoids and coumarin	Use as normal marmalade.
Tamari sauce	Health food shops	A type of soy sauce, made without using wheat	Use tamari sauce sparingly (since it is salty), to flavour stir-fried dishes. For dark soups and sauces use wheat-free miso (see above).
Tofu	Supermarkets and health food shops	A good source of protein made from soy – as good as eating meat but with added health benefits.	'Silken' tofu is good for liquidizing and making into mayonnaise, 'cheese'cake, or layering with vegetables etc. in oven-baked vegetable dishes. Ordinary firm tofu is best for cutting into cubes, dusting with brown rice flour and frying in oil. Can be marinated beforehand.

Phase II

Now you will be testing yourself for food allergies/intolerances. As explained in Chapter 2, a lot of fluid retention can be caused by odd reactions to common foods. But if these are foods you eat several times every day, you will never have the chance to realize that one or more of these may be linked with the fluid retention. The categories of food which most people eat very frequently are:

- Wheat (found in bread, flour, biscuits, sauces, puddings etc.)
- Dairy products (found in milk, cream, cheese, yoghurt, butter, and anything containing these)
- Yeast (found in alcoholic drinks, stock cubes and other savoury flavourings, gravy mix, bread and pizza)
- Egg (found in egg dishes, egg pasta, many brands of ice cream, desserts, batter, pancakes etc.)

If you lost a lot of fluid within a few days during Phase I of the Waterfall Diet, it is 90 per cent likely that you have an allergy or intolerance to one of these four foods. The only way to find out for sure is to reintroduce these foods into your diet one by one in a carefully controlled way. That is what Phase II is all about.

I do not recommend blood tests for discovering allergies. They are far less accurate because they are based on combining your blood with undigested food, and in the body your blood should never come into contact with undigested food. If it does, you would have a condition known as 'leaky gut syndrome', the treatment for which involves avoiding any foods which make you *feel* ill, and an intensive programme from a nutritional therapist to improve your digestion and heal the walls of your intestines.

Once you have completed all these tests, and have made a note of any foods that cause rapid weight gain or unpleasant symptoms, you can move on to Phase III.

Testing Procedure

Results

Week 1	In addition to your normal Phase I diet foods, eat egg-free wheat pasta, wheat flour or plain wheat crackers every day for five days, then stop. If you get any unpleasant reactions, such as headaches, sinus congestion or severe fatigue, or if your weight rises by several pounds during that time, you should stop before the five days is up – it is extremely likely that you have a wheat intolerance and need to continue avoiding wheat. Whether or not you experience a reaction, stop the wheat after five days and eat only Phase I diet foods for the next two days.
Week 2	Repeat what you did in Week 1, consuming cow's milk products, particularly fresh milk, cheese and yoghurt daily, instead of wheat. The procedure is exactly the same as for Week 1.
Week 3	Repeat what you did in Week 1, consuming eggs daily instead of wheat. If you do not want to eat a whole egg every day, make a two-egg omelette with plain egg and water, cook it very thinly, and eat a small strip each day for the test period.
Week 4	Repeat what you did in Week 1, consuming yeast daily instead of wheat. Buy a small jar of low-sodium yeast extract from a health food shop, and make it into a hot drink with half a teaspoon of yeast extract to a cup of boiling water. Drink this each day for the test period.

Phase III

This part of the Waterfall Diet is designed to be followed permanently, so that your fluid retention will remain controlled.

The 'Not Allowed' foods listed on p. 133 are no longer unconditionally forbidden. You may resume eating them, subject to two conditions:

- that you continue to avoid the specific foods which aggravate your particular *type* of fluid retention (see table on p. 166)

The Rules of Healthy Eating

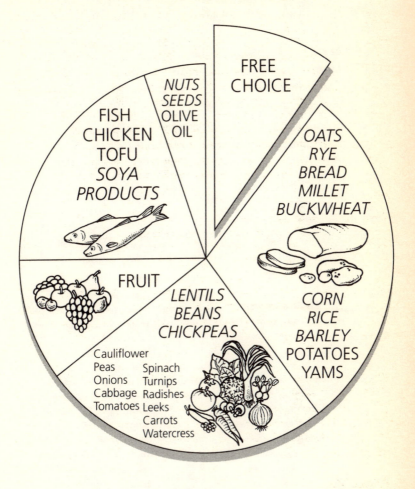

In Phase 3 of the Waterfall Diet, the foods you eat
should match the proportions shown on the plate above.
If you are a vegetarian, or if you do not eat fish or poultry
regularly, you should ensure that you eat a selection every
day of the vegetables, grains and other foods shown on the
plate in italics.

- 90 per cent of your diet should continue to consist of wholegrains and unrefined foods, fruits and vegetables and their juices, nuts and seeds, tofu and other soya products, and 'oily' fish.

So, for example, if Phase II of the diet shows that your type of fluid retention is allergic, and identifies dairy produce as the problem foods, then the 10 per cent of your food each day which is free choice can be anything you want, *except* for foods containing dairy produce. For instance you could have a fried dish, bread or sweet pastry, but not cow's milk with your cereals, cheese with your baked potatoes, or cow's milk yoghurt (please note that eggs are not dairy products).

Phase III Guidelines

Look at the tables on pp. 137 and 145 to remind you of the properties of the different foods mentioned below - which foods are high in fat, which ones help the liver, and so on.

If Your Fluid Retention Was Caused by	Foods to Avoid Completely	Foods to Keep to a Minimum	Foods to Emphasize	Other Useful Measures
Allergy	Any of the four foods tested in Phase II and found problematic	Alcohol, caffeine and artificial food additives	Quercetin-rich foods (e.g. apple peel, cabbage), magnesium- and B6-rich foods, foods which help the liver	Quercetin, magnesium, zinc and B vitamin supplements. Gut repair programme from a nutritional therapist
Protein	Nothing to be strictly rationed or emphasized, except for the general advice at the bottom of this table, since Phases I and II of the diet should have corrected your protein deficiency. Do not allow your protein-rich foods to drop to low levels again			HCl pepsin and digestive enzyme supplements, especially if your digestive ability has

			been impaired by long-term protein deficiency
Kidney Stress	Highly salted foods	Salt and sugary foods. Avoid eating a high-protein diet	Magnesium- and B6-rich foods, brazil nuts (for selenium)	Magnesium, vitamin B and selenium supplements
Prescription Medicines	Discuss with your doctor how necessary your medications are. Consider working with a nutritional therapist or other natural health practitioner so that in time perhaps you can be weaned off any currently unavoidable prescription medicines.			
Internal Pollution	Alcohol and caffeine	Foods high in saturated fat, sugar or refined flour, highly processed foods, fried foods, artificial food additives	Organically grown foods, filtered or bottled water, foods rich in natural fibre. Foods which help the liver, (see p. 137), turmeric, gelatine. Also ensure you consume adequate protein	Supplements of magnesium, taurine, reduced glutathione, N-acetyl cysteine, and the herbal extract silymarin. Add two crystals of Glaubers salts (sodium sulphate) to food daily. Avoid becoming constipated
Capillary or Lymphatic Problems	Meals containing no fruit or vegetables.	Coffee and alcohol. Foods high in saturated fat, sugar or refined flour, highly processed foods, fried foods	Vegetables and their juices. Flavonoid and coumarin-rich foods (see pp. 117 and 119)	Ginkgo biloba and horse-chestnut herbal supplements, buckwheat tea, clover

If Your Fluid Retention Was Caused by	Foods to Avoid Completely	Foods to Keep to a Minimum	Foods to Emphasize	Other Useful Measures
			especially citrus fruit and pith. Buckwheat	tea, dried clover flowers added to bath water. Exercise and massage
Vitamin and Mineral Deficiencies	Meals containing no fruits or vegetables	Foods high in saturated fat, sugar or refined flour, highly processed foods, fried foods	Wholegrains and unrefined foods. Fruits and vegetables and their juices, nuts and seeds, oily fish	Multivitamins and minerals, with extra zinc and magnesium
General	Meals containing no fruit or vegetables	Coffee, foods high in saturated fat, sugar or refined flour, highly processed foods, deep-fried foods, artificial food additives, salt and highly salted foods. If you are allowed alcohol, keep consumption low and preferably just red wine, which contains coumarin and beneficial flavonoids. Beer advertised as free of artificial additives would also be a good option	Wholegrains and unrefined foods. Fruit and vegetables and their juices, nuts and seeds, oily fish	Exercise, massage, multivitamins and minerals

Important note

If, after starting Phase III, you notice a return of any health problems such as joint pains, skin rashes or digestive problems, which had disappeared during Phase I, keep a diary of what you eat, what symptoms you experience and when you experience them. This will help you to identify what foods, such as occasional red meat, food additives and so on, might be responsible. If you are not able to identify the causes of your symptoms on your own, consider consulting a nutritional therapist (see Useful Addresses on p. 202).

Helpful advice

Fat in its natural form, as in butter, cream, red meat, olive oil or coconut oil, for example, is not damaging to your health unless eaten in excess (see p. 134). The difficulty is in knowing where the dividing line should be drawn. I often advise people to go ahead and use fat in their own cooking, because when you add it yourself you can control it. But if you buy ready-made burgers, pies, cakes, biscuits, desserts and so on the hidden fat can start to add up without you being aware of it. So you should always try to ration these foods (the table on p. 134 will show you more fully which foods are high-fat). For instance, meat legally sold as 'lean' can be up to 30 per cent fat, whether you can see the fat or not. Processed cheese is about 70 per cent fat.

Recipes

These recipes are suitable for all phases of the Waterfall Diet, and particularly for Phase I.

Breakfast recipes

Sheep's Milk or Soya Yoghurt With Apple Compote and Almonds

For one serving

Swirl 4 tablespoons sheep's milk or soya yoghurt into a generous serving of apple compote. Sprinkle liberally with toasted flaked almonds.

Sultana and Sunflower Seed Porridge with Soya Milk and Soya Cream

For one serving

Add 3 rounded dessertspoons of porridge oats or medium ground oatmeal to 1 mugful of unsweetened soya milk in a small, heavy-bottomed saucepan (enamelled cast iron if you have one). Bring to the boil, stirring constantly, then turn down the heat to a simmer and add 2 teaspoons sultanas and 2 teaspoons sunflower seeds. Keep stirring for a minute or two until it thickens. Add a little more soya milk when ready if you prefer a more runny porridge. Serve with a little soya cream poured over the top.

Variation
Soak the sultanas and sunflower seeds in the soya milk overnight before making the porridge.

Authentic Swiss Muesli with Flaked Nuts and Sweet Apricots

For one serving		
3 tablespoons medium or fine ground oatmeal	2 unsulphured dried apricots, chopped small
Water	
Soya or nut milk to taste	1 tablespoon flaked nuts

Did you know that the Swiss never eat muesli straight out of the packet? They know that raw grains should always be soaked overnight before eating them, because this breaks down mildly poisonous chemicals they contain, known as enzyme inhibitors, that can upset your intestines.

Soak the oatmeal overnight in the water. The amount of water you need will depend on how much the oatmeal can absorb – about three times its volume for medium oatmeal, and more for fine oatmeal. If you find after an hour or so that the mixture has become too solid, add more water. No milk is necessary since the oats create their own milk. In the morning check the consistency and add a little soya or nut milk if you wish, to achieve your preferred consistency. If you use fine oatmeal, the result will be very creamy. Stir in the dried apricot pieces and sprinkle with flaked nuts.

Note
Dried apricots are orange in colour if treated with sulphur dioxide. This additive is an intestinal irritant and can cause bloating and gas. Unsulphured apricots (from health food shops) are dark brown and much sweeter in flavour.

Avocado 'Smoothie' with Soya Milk, Banana and Strawberries

FOR 2 SERVINGS
Liquidize an avocado with $\frac{3}{4}$ pint (500 ml) soya milk, half a banana and a handful of strawberries. Drink immediately.

Soups and salads

Cream of Brussels Sprout, Broccoli, Celery or Cauliflower Soup

FOR 6 SERVINGS

1 medium head broccoli
or celery or small head
cauliflower, or 8 oz
(225 g) Brussels sprouts
1 large potato
1 large onion

$1\frac{1}{2}$ pints (1 litre) water
$\frac{1}{4}$ teaspoon mixed dried
herbs
1 teaspoon potassium salt
Freshly ground black
pepper to taste
3 tablespoons soya cream

If using broccoli, peel the stalk first. Chop all the vegetables into smallish pieces, then place in a pan with the water and salt, cover, bring to the boil and simmer until soft (about 20 minutes).

Using a slotted spoon, remove one spoonful of the vegetable pieces and reserve. Liquidize the remainder in the pan with a hand blender. Return the reserved pieces to the pan, add the herbs, salt and pepper and stir in the soya cream.

Chunky Winter Vegetable Soup with Marrowfat Peas

Use the above basic recipe, but replace the main ingredients with 2 large carrots, 1 leek and 1 small white turnip. After liquidizing the soup, add a few handfuls of cooked marrowfat peas and a handful of chopped parsley.

Lentil Soup with Miso, Celery and Onion

FOR 6 SERVINGS

½ pint (275 ml) dried brown, red or Puy lentils
1 large onion, chopped
6 sticks celery, chopped
1½ pints (1 litre) water

1 heaped tablespoon wheat-free miso paste
1 tablespoon unsalted tomato puree (optional)
¼ teaspoon mixed dried herbs
Pinch of cayenne pepper

Simmer all the ingredients together until cooked (about 30 minutes). Remove one spoonful, thicken the rest by liquidizing with a hand blender, then return the reserved spoonful to the pan.

Shredded White Cabbage with Grated Carrot in Yoghurt and Mustard Vinaigrette

FOR 1 SERVING

1 large handful finely shredded raw white cabbage
1 handful coarsely grated raw carrot
1 tablespoon dry roasted unsalted peanuts, crushed (optional)
2 tablespoons extra virgin olive oil

1 tablespoon lemon juice
½ teaspoon English mustard
1 tablespoon soya yoghurt
Pinch of potassium salt
Freshly ground black pepper to taste

Combine the cabbage and carrot in a bowl, plus the peanuts if you are using them. Whip the oil, lemon juice, mustard, yoghurt and seasonings together in a small dish and pour over the vegetable mixure.

Broccoli in Vinaigrette with Sliced Spring Onion

FOR 3 SERVINGS 1 spring onion (scallion), French dressing to taste
finely sliced 1 medium head of
broccoli

Mix the onion with the dressing. Cut the head off the broccoli
stem. Peel the stem (or save it for juicing) and separate the head
into small florets. Steam the florets for 12–15 minutes or until just
tender. Pour the French dressing and spring onion mixture over
it, and gently turn the florets until the dressing is evenly distrib-
uted. Eat warm or cold – try it served on a bed of alfalfa sprouts.

Tomato Slices on a Bed of Alfalfa Sprouts and Grated Radish with French Dressing and Tofu Mayonnaise

FOR 1 SERVING 1 large handful alfalfa 3 tablespoons French
sprouts dressing
1 large handful grated 1 tablespoon tofu
mooli radish mayonnaise
1 beef tomato, sliced (see recipe on p. 191)

Place the alfalfa sprouts in a dish or lunch box, cover with
grated radish and tomato slices, pour French dressing over them,
then top with a dollop of tofu mayonnaise.

Beetroot and Orange Salad

FOR 2 GENEROUS
SERVINGS

1 raw beetroot, peeled and grated, *or* 1 cooked beetroot, chopped
½ orange, lightly peeled (to keep some white pith) and sliced
½ eating apple, chopped
8 black grapes, halved with seeds removed

1 stick celery, chopped
1 spring onion (scallion), sliced
6–8 freshly shelled walnuts chopped into fairly large pieces
4–6 sprigs watercress, roughly chopped

DRESSING:

The juice of ½ an orange (about 2 tablespoons)
1 dessertspoon olive oil

Generous pinch of mixed dried herbs
Potassium salt
Freshly ground black pepper

Prepare the dressing by mixing the orange juice with the olive oil and then whisking with a fork. Add the herbs, salt and black pepper. Place the prepared fruit and vegetables and place in a salad dish. Pour the dressing over and serve immediately.

Main dishes

Mediterranean Squid with Onions and Brown Rice

This garlic-rich dish is thoroughly cooked, which removes both the pungency and smell of garlic. Your breath will not smell of garlic after eating it!

FOR 2 SERVINGS

1 large squid
4 tablespoons olive oil
1 whole bulb garlic, peeled and crushed
2 large onions, chopped
2 cans chopped Italian plum tomatoes

1 tablespoon unsalted tomato puree
1 tablespoon chopped parsley *or* 1 teaspoon dried parsley
$\frac{1}{2}$ teaspoon potassium salt
Cayenne pepper to taste

Clean the squid (or ask the fishmonger to do it for you), by removing the 'quill' and insides and discarding everything except the body, fins and tentacle meat. Cut into bite-size pieces, rinse and mop dry with kitchen paper. Heat the oil in a large, heavy-bottomed saucepan or pressure cooker, and gently cook the onions until they begin to soften, stirring occasionally. Add the garlic, stir for another minute and then add the squid pieces, turning up the heat as you do so. Stir-fry the ingredients for another minute and then add the tomatoes and tomato puree. Stir thoroughly, bring to the boil, then turn the heat down very low, cover the pan and simmer gently for 1 hour. (If using a pressure cooker, bring to full steam, then cook for 20 minutes.) Thicken the sauce by turning up the heat a little, removing the lid and continuing to cook with the lid off, stirring occasionally, until reduced to a thick, glossy consistency. Add the parsley and seasoning. Serve with brown rice and a green salad.

The Quickest, Healthiest Kedgeree Ever

FOR 1 SERVING

4 oz (110 g) cod *or* haddock *or* salmon fillet, skinned
2 tablespoons extra virgin olive oil
4 tablespoons chopped mixed frozen vegetables (e.g. carrots and red sweet peppers diced small, peas, sweetcorn)

Few drops Tabasco sauce
1 teaspoon tamari sauce
1 portion cooked brown rice
1 tablespoon mushroom pieces which have been fried in olive oil
2 tablespoons water
1 teaspoon chopped fresh parsley

Place the fish in a pan with enough water to come halfway up the fish. Bring to the boil, then cover and simmer very gently for 5 minutes, or until the fish flakes easily. Meanwhile heat the olive oil in a heavy-bottomed saucepan, or preferably a wok, and add the frozen vegetables. Stir-fry over medium heat until they have defrosted and any water has evaporated. Then add the Tabasco and tamari sauce, followed by the rice and mushrooms and stir in with the vegetables. Turn the heat down very low, sprinkle in the water and cover. While the rice is heating, drain the fish and separate into flakes. By now the rice should be hot. Remove from the heat and add the fish flakes, folding them into the rice very gently so that they do not break. Serve sprinkled with parsley.

Variations
For a more risotto-like texture you could stir in some warm soya cream before adding the fish. Or for a tomato flavour, add some tomato puree along with the Tabasco and tamari sauce.

Spicy Bean and Vegetable Rosti

For 2 servings

9 oz (250 g) cooked borlotti beans *or* black-eyed beans
½ small onion, finely chopped or grated
1 stick celery, finely chopped

½ tablespoon Sojasun soya yoghurt

1 tablespoon unsalted tomato purée
2 rounded teaspoons dried parsley
½ teaspoon curry powder
Potassium salt
Freshly ground black pepper
3 medium potatoes
Extra virgin olive oil for cooking

Mash the beans roughly with a fork, and mix with the remaining ingredients except the olive oil and potato. Form the bean mixture into six patties. Peel and grate the potato and squeeze out the excess water with your hands. Cover both sides of each bean patty with grated potato and press gently between your hands. The potato will create quite a ragged covering, but this will adhere to the mixture when you start to cook the patties. Gently heat a little oil in a heavy-bottomed frying pan. Slide a spatula under each rosti to transfer it to the pan, and cook gently in batches of 2 or 3 for 5–8 minutes each side or until the potato is brown and crisp. Serve immediately with a mixed salad and a spoonful of soya yoghurt garnished with chopped coriander leaves.

Vegetable and Lentil Pasties

FOR 2 LARGE PASTIES

1 small onion, finely chopped
Extra virgin olive oil
2 oz (50 g) shredded cabbage
2 oz (50 g) frozen peas
2 oz (50 g) cooked Puy lentils (small green lentils)
1 tablespoon unsalted tomato purée
1 dessertspoon soya yoghurt
$\frac{1}{2}$ teaspoon dried oregano
Generous pinch of mixed dried herbs
Freshly grated nutmeg
Potassium salt
Freshly ground black pepper
1 teaspoon soya flour
4 teaspoons water
Sesame seeds
1 quantity of the Healthiest Pastry In The World (see recipe on p. 193)

Preheat the oven to 200°C/400°F/gas mark 6. Gently cook the onions in a little olive oil until beginning to brown. Add the cabbage, peas and lentils. Cook for 2–3 minutes. Add the tomato purée, soya yoghurt, herbs, nutmeg, salt and pepper. Set to one side.

Divide the pastry dough into two pieces. Roll out on a floured board, place a tea plate over the top and trim round with a knife so that you have a perfect round of dough. Brush a little cold water around the edge of the circle of pastry. Place some of the filling in the middle and fold in half to create a semi-circle. Seal the edges by pressing with a fork or the tip of a knife. Make two small incisions with a knife in the top of the pasty to allow steam to escape. Repeat until you have used all the ingredients.

To make a glaze, mix the soya flour with the 4 teaspoons water. Brush on to each pasty and sprinkle with sesame seeds. Place the pasties on an oiled baking tray and bake for approximately 20–25 minutes or until golden brown.

Twice-baked Potatoes

FOR 2 SERVINGS

2 baking potatoes, well scrubbed

2 tablespoons hummus (see recipe on p. 189)

1 tablespoon finely chopped onion

1 spring onion, finely sliced

1 stick celery, finely chopped

Preheat the oven to 200°C/400°F/gas mark 6. Bake the potatoes until they feel soft when you squeeze them. Remove from the oven and slice in half lengthways. Scoop out the flesh, leaving the skins intact. Combine the potato, hummus, onion, spring onion and celery, mixing well, and then pile into the potato skin halves. Place on an ovenproof dish and return to the oven. Bake for another 20 minutes or until the potato mixture is beginning to brown. Serve with beetroot and orange salad.

Red Thai Curry with Pan-Fried Tofu

FOR 1 SERVING

3 thick slices from a block of firm tofu
Potassium salt
Cayenne pepper
Groundnut oil for frying
$\frac{1}{4}$ pint (150 ml) water
2 teaspoons red Thai curry paste (more if you like it stronger)

$\frac{1}{2}$ inch (1 cm) piece cut from a block of creamed coconut
$\frac{1}{2}$ cup mixed frozen vegetables (e.g. carrots and red sweet peppers diced small, peas, sweetcorn)
1 portion uncooked vermicelli rice noodles or 1 portion cooked brown rice

Cut the tofu into bite-size pieces, pat dry with kitchen paper and sprinkle with salt and cayenne pepper. Heat the oil to a depth of $\frac{1}{4}$ inch (.5 cm) in a frying pan. When hot enough for the tofu to sizzle when added, carefully put the pieces in the pan and fry on each side for 1–2 minutes or until golden. Drain on kitchen paper.

Heat the water in a pan. Add the curry paste and coconut cream, stirring until dissolved. Add the frozen vegetables, cover the pan and simmer for a few minutes.

Place the vermicelli rice noodles in a bowl. Boil a kettleful of water and pour the water generously over the noodles, leaving them plenty of room to swell. Leave for 4 minutes, then run a little cold water into the bowl before draining the noodles thoroughly in a large sieve. If using rice, heat the rice in a tightly lidded pan over a low heat with a tablespoon of water.

When the vegetables are heated through, stir in the fried tofu pieces and coat with the sauce. Serve the rice or noodles with the vegetables and tofu on top and a little of the sauce spooned over.

Hawaiian Tofu Kebabs

FOR 2 SERVINGS

1 stick celery cut into 8 x 1 inch (2 cm) pieces
½ red pepper cut into 8 pieces
½ yellow or orange pepper cut into 8 pieces
8 cherry tomatoes

8 button mushrooms
8 chunks of fresh pineapple or canned pineapple in juice (not syrup)
1 packet firm tofu, cut into 16 cubes
sesame seeds (optional)

MARINADE:

½ teaspoon miso
3 fl oz (75 ml) pineapple juice, either extracted from fresh pineapple or taken from the can
2 tablespoons fresh orange juice

1 small clove garlic, crushed
1 pinch ground ginger
½ dessertspoon olive oil
2–3 drops tamari sauce
Freshly ground black pepper

To make the marinade, dissolve the miso paste in a little pineapple juice, then combine with the remaining marinade ingredients in a large bowl. Place the vegetables, pineapple and tofu in a large, shallow dish. Pour the marinade over the top and store in the fridge for at least one hour. Stir gently from time to time and spoon the marinade over the pieces of fruit, vegetable and tofu, making sure they are all well covered.

Thread the vegetables, pineapple and tofu chunks on to metal skewers. Pour the marinade into a saucepan and simmer over medium heat until reduced and slightly thickened. Preheat the grill on medium heat. Balance the threaded skewers over a shallow dish and either brush the thickened marinade on to each piece or drizzle it over with a spoon. Sprinkle with sesame seeds if liked, and grill the kebabs until the vegetables are tender and beginning to brown. Turn the skewers regularly to ensure the kebabs are browned on each side.

Serve on a bed of long grain brown rice, with a mixed salad and a side dish of soya yoghurt combined with finely chopped cucumber and fresh mint.

Nutty Mushroom Bake

In this recipe a cup is an ordinary teacup

FOR 3–4 SERVINGS

1 onion, quartered
2 sticks celery, roughly cut into segments
1 small green pepper, cut into 8 pieces
4 tablespoons olive oil
1 medium carrot, grated
4 oz (125 g) mushrooms, diced

2 oz (50 g) walnuts, coarsely ground in food processor
A few leaves of fresh basil, chopped
Freshly ground black pepper to taste
tamari sauce
2 cups cooked brown rice

Preheat the oven to 400°F/200°C/gas mark 6.

Grease a loaf tin. Process the onion, celery and green pepper together in a food processor until finely chopped. Place a large, heavy-bottomed saucepan, or preferably a wok, over a medium-high heat, and when hot, add 2 tablespoons olive oil, followed by the onion, celery and green pepper mixture and the grated carrot. Stir-fry for five minutes until the mixture begins to soften, then take off the heat and transfer the contents to a bowl.

Clean and dry the pan then replace over a medium-high heat and add the diced mushrooms. Stir-fry without oil for a minute to dry them out a little, then add the oil and continue to stir-fry until golden brown.

Take off the heat, replace the vegetables in the pan, and mix in the chopped walnuts, basil, pepper and a few dashes of tamari sauce. Finally fold the rice grains in gently, ensuring that they do not break up. Transfer the contents to a loaf tin, smooth down evenly with a fork, cover with foil and bake for about 40 minutes. Serve with tomato slices on a bed of alfalfa sprouts and grated radish, with french dressing and tofu mayonnaise (see p. 174).

Variations
Use cooked buckwheat or millet instead of brown rice, or include a tablespoon of wild rice.

Dessert recipes

Fresh Fruit Compote or Jelly

Fresh or frozen sweet fruit: berries, cherries, apricots, peaches, apples etc.
Gelatine or vegetarian gelling product (optional)

Red grape juice or orange juice (optional)
Handful of raisins and a few drops of lemon juice (if using apples)

If using frozen fruit allow to defrost first. Place the fruits or fruit pieces in an ovenproof dish in a medium oven for 25 minutes or until they split and the juices run. Serve hot or cold, or turn into fruit jelly by stirring in some gelatine or vegetarian gelling product dissolved in warm water, red grape juice or orange juice before cooling. (Use the directions on the packet to gauge the amount of gelling product required.) If extra sweetening is needed, use a teaspoon of date purée (see p. 192).

If using apples, select a naturally sweet variety. Cut into quarters and remove the core, then cut into small pieces or slices, placing the pieces in a bowl of cold water with lemon juice added to prevent them turning brown before they are cooked. Mix with a handful of raisins before placing in an ovenproof dish and cooking as described above.

Serve with soya yoghurt or soya cream.

In Phase III of the diet, if you are allowed alcohol you can add some red wine such as Lambrusco (a sweet Italian low-alcohol sparkling wine) to the compote before cooking. The wine can also be made into jelly.

Date and Chestnut Dream

Allow 4–5 unsweetened canned chestnuts for each serving (or boil fresh chestnuts until soft and shell them yourself), plus 1 rounded tablespoon date purée (see recipe on p. 192) and up to $\frac{1}{4}$ pint (150 ml) soya cream. Mash the chestnuts with a fork, then mix with the date purée and most of the soya cream. Whizz with a blender until the mixture has the consistency of thick cream. Serve in glass dishes with the remaining soya cream poured on top and decorate with a little grated bitter chocolate and a black cherry.

Chocolate Banana Cream Boats

INGREDIENTS FOR 6 SERVINGS	1 x 9oz (250 g) pack Sanchi organic tofu 8 bananas, peeled 2 teaspoons cocoa powder	2 handfuls sunflower seeds A few tablespoons soya milk
TO GARNISH	pieces of fruit (canned mandarin orange segments, cherries, or	chopped peach) or a sprig of mint, and flaked nuts.

This brand of tofu is an extra firm silken tofu (see p. 162) variety and has a smooth, creamy texture. Roughly chop the tofu and two of the bananas, then whizz in a blender with the cocoa powder, sunflower seeds and some of the soya milk until the mixture looks creamy. Add a little more soya milk if the cream is too thick.

Cut the remaining six bananas lengthwise into halves and place in pairs on a serving dish. Dollop each pair with the chocolate banana cream and slightly press together to make a 'boat' shape. Decorate with your chosen garnish and serve immediately.

You could also use the chocolate banana cream as a topping for the blinis in the next recipe.

Black Forest Blinis

MAKES 16 BLINIS
Blinis:

4 oz (110 g) buckwheat flour	2 tablespoons raisins
1 oz (25 g) soya flour	8 fl oz (225 ml) diluted soya milk
2 teaspoons ground cinnamon	2 tablespoon soya yoghurt or liquidized silken tofu
1 teaspoon potassium baking powder	Olive or groundnut oil for cooking

Topping

Sugar-free black cherry jam	Soya yoghurt
	A little grated bitter chocolate

To make the blinis, mix together the dry ingredients. Slowly add the diluted soya milk to make a thick, pourable batter. Stir in the soya yoghurt or liquidized silken tofu and beat well with a wooden spoon. If necessary add more liquid to achieve the right consistency, which should be similar to the batter used for 'drop scones': a spoonful dropped in the pan should spread out by itself to a thickness of about $\frac{1}{4}$ inch ($\frac{1}{2}$ cm). Heat a heavy-bottomed frying pan on medium heat and wipe over with a wad of kitchen paper dipped in a little oil. Drop tablespoonfuls of the mixture into the hot pan and cook until small holes appear in the batter. Flip over, using a metal spatula, and cook the second side for about the same length of time. Re-oil the pan between each batch. The blinis should be light, fluffy and golden brown on the outside. Serve warm, spread with the black cherry jam and a teaspoon of soya yoghurt. Sprinkle with the grated bitter chocolate.

Topping Variations
- A teaspoon of soya yoghurt sprinkled with toasted sesame seeds and topped with sliced fresh pear.
- A teaspoon of banana cream (see previous recipe).

- Apple and raisin compote or sugar-free marmalade plus a dollop of soya yoghurt.

Brown Rice Pudding

FOR 4 SERVINGS

4 oz (110 g) short grain brown rice, which has been soaked overnight in water and then drained
1 litre carton soya milk

1 small knob creamed coconut
1 handful raisins
1 tablespoon chopped almonds, *or* pulp from making almond milk

Place all the ingredients in a heavy-bottomed saucepan (enamelled cast iron is best) and bring to a gentle simmer, stirring until the creamed coconut has dissolved. Put a heat diffuser under the pan and leave covered on the lowest setting for 2 hours. Check occasionally to ensure that the rice pudding is not beginning to stick to the bottom of the pan, and stir gently if necessary. Alternatively, cook the pudding for the same time in a greased ovenproof dish in an oven preheated to 175°C/325°F or gas mark 3.

Sultana and Coconut Cheesecake Ramekins

MAKES 3 RAMEKINS

1oz (25 g) sultanas
½oz (10 g) chopped mixed nuts
½oz (10 g) oatflakes
½oz (10 g) dessicated coconut
½oz (10 g) gelatine

juice of 1 orange
1 teaspoon natural vanilla extract
1 x 9 oz (250 g) pack of organic Sanchi tofu (this is an extra firm silken tofu)

Put the sultanas in a small saucepan with four tablespoons of water. Bring to the boil and simmer very gently for 10 minutes, adding a little more water if necessary to prevent them from boiling dry. Meanwhile, lightly oil the inside of three ramekins or small moulds (about $3\frac{1}{2}$ inches/9 cm) in diameter. Toast the chopped mixed nuts and oatflakes in a frying pan over a medium heat for five minutes until beginning to brown. Take off the heat and stir in the dessicated coconut. Divide this mixture between the ramekins and press down firmly.

Remove the sultanas from the heat. Sprinkle the gelatine on to four tablespoons of cold water in a heat-proof bowl or double-boiler, and mix thoroughly, ensuring there are no lumps. Once the mixture has turned into a thick paste, place the dish in or over a pan of boiling water. Stir the gelatine as it dissolves. When fully dissolved, stir in the sultanas, orange juice and vanilla essence.

Using a hand blender, whizz this mixture into the tofu until smooth and creamy, then spoon into the ramekin dishes. Chill until set. To turn out, stand the ramekin dishes in hot water for a minute, then turn upside-down.

Snack recipes

Carolyn's Special Spicy Carrot Cake

In this recipe a cup means an ordinary teacup

1 cup dates (stoned)	$1\frac{3}{4}$ cups spelt flour
$1\frac{1}{4}$ cups water	$\frac{1}{4}$ cup soya flour
$\frac{3}{4}$ cup raisins	2 teaspoons potassium
2 large carrots, finely	baking powder
grated	1 cup chopped hazelnuts
2 teaspoons mixed spice	

Simmer the dates, water, raisins, carrots and spices together in a pan for 5 minutes. Cover and allow to stand overnight. Next day preheat the oven to 170°C/325°F/Gas Mark 3. Oil a 6–7 inch (15–18 cm) cake tin and line with greaseproof paper. Combine the flours and baking powder and add them and the hazelnuts to the carrot mixture, mixing well. Bake for $1\frac{1}{2}$–2 hours in the centre of the oven. The cake is ready when a skewer comes out clean. Leave for a few minutes in the tin, them turn out on a wire rack to finish cooling.

Derbyshire Oatcakes

These delicious pancake-like oatcakes are usually made with a yeast batter but this recipe, using a yoghurt-based mixture, is just as good and produces a lovely nutty texture. They can be eaten with savoury or sweet accompaniments or just on their own, as an alternative to bread or crackers

4 oz (110 g) medium oatmeal
4 oz (110 g) spelt flour
5 fl oz (150 ml) (tepid) soya milk
$\frac{1}{2}$ pint (275 ml) (tepid) water

2 tablespoons soya yoghurt or liquidized silken tofu
2 teaspoons potassium baking powder

Mix the oatmeal and flour together in a large mixing bowl. Gradually stir in the milk, water and yoghurt or liquidized silken tofu with a large wooden spoon, then beat well to produce a smooth, thick batter. Leave covered for 1 hour (or overnight if you will be eating the oatcakes for breakfast). Just before cooking, stir in the baking powder.

Heat a large, heavy-bottomed frying pan. Lightly wipe the surface of the hot pan with a wad of kitchen paper dipped into a little oil. Using a ladle or small cup, pour enough batter into the pan to just cover the bottom. Immediately tilt and turn the pan so that the batter runs to the edge of the pan, forming a pancake shape. Cook the oatcake on a medium heat for about a minute or until it will leave the pan cleanly and is beginning to brown. Slide a metal spatula underneath and flip it over. Cook the second side for about the same time.

Continue with the rest of the batter, stacking the cooked oatcakes on a plate. Stir the batter regularly to keep the pouring consistency. Oil the pan again between each batch.

If the oatcakes are not for eating immediately, stack them on a plate, separated by a layer of absorbent kitchen paper, as you cook them. Once cool, they will keep for a few days in the fridge and need only be briefly heated under the grill before eating. If freezing the oatcakes, first place them in the freezer individually, i.e. not in a stack, otherwise they will stick together as they freeze. They can be toasted straight from the freezer.

Hummus

In this recipe a cup means an ordinary teacup

FOR 4 SERVINGS

1½ cups freshly cooked chick peas

½ cup cooking liquid from the chick peas

2 heaped tablespoons sesame seeds

4 tablespoons extra virgin olive oil

1 tablespoon lemon juice

1 clove garlic, crushed

½ teaspoon potassium salt

Cayenne pepper to taste

Blend all the ingredients together in a food processor, adding more cooking liquid if necessary, until the mixture achieves the consistency of a thick dip. Use as a dip for crudités or slit open a griddle bread (see recipe on p. 194) and stuff with hummus mixed with alfalfa sprouts, peanuts, green pepper strips and grated radish.

Roasted Vegetable Pissaladière

FOR 1 SERVING

Extra virgin olive oil
½ yellow pepper, cut into chunks
1 fresh ripe tomato, quartered
5–6 button mushrooms, sliced
1 small onion, thinly sliced
1 round of griddle bread

dough (uncooked, see recipe on p. 194)
Tomato purée
6 black olives (choose a low-salt variety), pitted and halved
Mixed herbs
Freshly ground black pepper

Preheat the oven to 200°C/400°F/gas mark 6. Rub a little olive oil on a roasting tray. Place the prepared vegetables on the tray and drizzle a few drops of olive oil over them. Roast for about 10 minutes or until the vegetables are beginning to soften and brown. Oil a small, shallow ovenproof dish and place the dough round in the base. Spread a little tomato purée on the dough and pile the roasted vegetables on top. Garnish with the black olive halves and dot a little more tomato purée around the vegetables. Sprinkle with mixed herbs and a little black pepper. Bake for 15–20 minutes. Check that the dough base is cooked through and then serve immediately.

Fruity Almond Cookies

So sweet, no-one will realize they're made without sugar!

MAKES 18–20

4 oz (110 g) unsulphured dried apricots
4 oz (110 g) ground almonds
2 oz (50 g) chopped mixed nuts

2 oz (50 g) mixed dried fruit with peel
4 oz (50g) soya flour
1 level teaspoon potassium baking powder
1 teaspoon natural vanilla essence

Preheat the oven to 350°F/180°C/gas mark 4. Lightly oil a baking sheet. Dice the dried apricots, place them in a small saucepan and just cover with water. Bring to the boil and simmer very gently for 30 minutes. Add a little more water if necessary to prevent them drying out. Mix the dry ingredients together.

Once the apricots are cooked, purée them with a hand blender, adding a little more water if necessary to obtain a thick, smooth purée. Stir in the vanilla essence, then mix into the dry ingredients. Incorporate thoroughly, to achieve a thick, stiff paste. Roll the paste into two long sausage shapes. Divide each roll into 10 segments. Roll each segment into a ball with your hands, press your hands together to flatten it, and place it on the baking sheet. Bake in the preheated oven for 20 minutes. If the cookies become too soft after a day or two, they can be restored by gently warming under the grill.

Miscellaneous recipes

Basic French Dressing (Vinaigrette)

$\frac{1}{4}$ pint (150 ml) extra
   virgin olive oil
2 fl oz (55 ml) wine
   vinegar *or* cider vinegar
$\frac{1}{4}$ teaspoon potassium salt
Pinch of mixed dried
   herbs

$\frac{1}{4}$ teaspoon English
   mustard (optional)
Freshly ground black
   pepper to taste

Whisk the ingredients together until thick and store in the fridge in a screw top jar. Shake vigorously before use.

Tofu Mayonnaise

$\frac{1}{2}$ packet soft silken tofu
1 teaspoon lemon juice
Pinch of potassium salt

2 fl oz (55 ml) extra
   virgin olive oil
Freshly ground black
   pepper to taste

Liquidize the first three ingredients, then whizz in the olive oil a little at a time. Stir in ground black pepper.

Variation:
You could also flavour this recipe with a teaspoon of mustard powder.

Date Purée

This recipe is used for sweetening or can be mixed with soya cream for a delicious accompaniment to desserts. Put a generous handful of dried stoned dates in a small, heavy-bottomed saucepan (ideally enamelled cast iron) and just cover with water. Bring to the boil, then simmer very gently, covered, for about 10 minutes or until soft and mushy. The dates should have absorbed most of the water. If any remains, boil it away fast until there is no more than a tablespoon or two of liquid left in the pan. Remove the pan from the heat and purée the dates with a hand blender.

Home-made Soya Yoghurt

No special equipment is needed, but if you do have a yoghurt maker it will work just as well with soya milk as with cow's milk. Otherwise use a bowl with a well-fitting lid or a wide-necked thermos flask. Make sure everything is sterilized before use as any bacteria on the utensils will compete with the yoghurt-making bacteria and the results will be disappointing.

1 500 ml carton unsweetened soya milk
2 tablespoons starter culture (either your own previously made soya yoghurt, or a commercial brand such as Sojasun)

Boil the soya milk, then pour into a clean bowl, thermos flask or yoghurt maker. Allow to cool to blood heat (around 30 minutes). If you have a yoghurt or cooking thermometer, the temperature should be about 98°F/37°C; if not, a clean finger dipped into the milk works just as well – it should feel 'comfortable' at blood heat.

Stir the starter into the milk and whisk briefly. If using the yoghurt maker, follow the manufacturer's instructions. Otherwise, if using a bowl, place the lid firmly on top and wrap securely in a towel or tea cosy to retain the heat. Place in a warm part of the kitchen such as above the fridge, or in a warm airing cupboard, for 12 hours. If using a thermos flask, simply tighten the screw top and leave for 12 hours. Finally, empty into a lidded container and keep refrigerated until use.

The consistency of home-made soya yoghurt is variable. Sometimes it can be quite runny and other times well set. If yours turns out to be runny, beat it well with a clean spoon (keeping it in the receptacle you made it in), replace the lid, and put it in the fridge. After a few hours it should have thickened a little. Runny yoghurt can still be used for soups, casseroles, muesli etc.

The Healthiest Pastry in the World

> 4 oz (110 g) spelt flour
> 2 oz (50 g) full-fat soya flour
> Approx 3 $\frac{1}{2}$ fl oz (generous 100 ml) cold water

Sift the spelt flour into a mixing bowl. Add the soya flour and mix well with a fork. Gradually add enough cold water to make a firm dough. Knead very lightly and place in a polythene bag. Store in the fridge for at least 1 hour. Roll out on a floured board and use as required.

Griddle Bread

This is a versatile chapatti-type bread that can be used as a pizza base, an accompaniment to curry, a base for open sandwiches, or split open and stuffed like pitta bread with a variety of fillings.

To make about 9 breads

10 oz (275 g) spelt flour	Scant teaspoon warm
2 tablespoons soya	water
yoghurt	

Preheat a dry griddle pan or cast-iron frying pan on a moderate heat for about 2 minutes. Add the yoghurt and warm water to the flour and mix to a soft, pliable dough. Turn out on to a well-floured board and knead lightly, adding more flour if necessary to prevent sticking. Break off egg-sized pieces of dough, and using more flour, roll out into rounds measuring about 6 inch (15 cm) in diameter and $\frac{1}{4}$ inch (0.5 cm) thick. Add more flour to the board as necessary and dust each round with a little flour before cooking.

When the pan is hot, place one or two rounds of dough on it and cook for $1\frac{1}{2}$ minutes on each side, or until small brown spots appear. To complete the cooking, place the breads in a toaster or under a preheated grill. The breads should puff up. Don't leave them to cook for too long at this stage or they will become hard. Serve immediately.

The dough will keep overnight if covered and stored in the fridge. It does tend to become stickier with keeping, so extra flour should be kneaded in before rolling out.

To Freeze: Allow the breads to cool after cooking on the griddle pan, and omit the toasting/grilling stage. Place in polythene freezer bags before freezing. To use, simply toast or grill the breads from frozen.

Variations: Make as above to the rolling-out stage. Brush one side of each dough round with soya milk or water. Sprinkle generously with any combination of sesame seeds, sunflower seeds and linseeds, and press the seeds into the dough with the palm of your hand or the rolling pin. Cook as above.

Brown Rice

Wash thoroughly, then soak overnight in twice its volume of filtered water. Use the same water for cooking. Bring to the boil, then cover tightly and simmer on the lowest possible heat for 20 minutes. If the water has not all been absorbed, drain away the excess (or save it for adding to soup, as it is very rich in vitamins). Leave the rice in the covered saucepan away from the heat for 5 minutes, after which it is ready to serve.

Once cold, brown rice can be spread out on an oiled baking tray, frozen, then crumbled into grains and bagged for the freezer.

Cooking Dried Beans and Peas

Haricot, kidney, borlotti or flageoli beans, black-eyed beans, butter beans, chick peas, marrowfat peas and split peas should all be soaked in water before use. Cover with four times their volume in boiling filtered water and leave overnight. Throw away the soaking water. Cover the beans with fresh water in a pressure cooker, bring to full steam and cook for 3–8 minutes, depending on size. Pressure-cooking breaks down the poisonous lectins found in raw beans. If you do not have a pressure cooker, boil them fast for at least 10 minutes before simmering or slow-cooking – conventional boiling may take up to 2 hours to soften them, depending on age and size.

To freeze, allow to cool and follow the same procedure as for frozen brown rice.

Drinks

It is best to drink home-made juices the same day you make them.

Home-made Apple, Celery, Parsley and Radish Juice

For 1 serving

1 large sweet apple, unpeeled and organic if possible
2 sticks celery
1 bunch parsley

2 inch (5 cm) segment of mooli radish
Small piece of lemon (optional – you may find that it helps the flavour) including peel

Wash the ingredients, cut them into chunks and put them through a juice extractor. Stir, and leave to stand for 20 minutes to break down the peppery taste of the radish before drinking.

Beetroot, Celery and Lemon Juice

Combine equal quantities of bottled beetroot juice and home-made celery juice (made from fresh celery with a juice extractor). Flavour with a little fresh lemon juice to taste.

If you juice your own raw beetroot, it will be very strong and only a little is required. It must be left to stand for 20 minutes before drinking or else it will have a very peppery taste.

Home-made Broccoli Stem and Sharp Apple Juice

Broccoli juice is very sweet, which is why it is good mixed with a fairly sharp apple juice. Simply cut the broccoli stems and apples into chunks and feed into your juice extractor in the proportions you prefer. You may need to experiment a little. If necessary, add a little lemon juice to disguise the broccoli flavour.

Carrot and Orange Juice

This is a lovely sweet combination. Simply mix half carrot and half orange juice together. If you do not have a juice extractor, buy juices and use your liquidizer to whizz in a piece of orange peel with the pith still attached. Buy unwaxed oranges if you can find them.

Flavonoid-rich Orange Juice

Liquidize a piece of fresh orange (preferably unwaxed) with pith and peel into a glass of normal orange juice. This will contain a far larger quantity of flavonoids than you could get in a flavonoid supplement pill!

Home-made Clover Tea

Clover grows almost anywhere there is long grass. Pick the flowers in a clean spot (not the roadside, which may be contaminated with dust from car exhausts) and dry them in the sun to bring out the coumarin, then steep in boiling water for 5 minutes, strain and drink the liquid. You could also add some grated ginger, comfrey tea leaves, chamomile, or orange or lemon zest. Some specialist herbal suppliers sell dried clover flowers.

Almond Milk

This delicious drink is made by soaking a large handful of blanched almonds in 1 pint (570 ml) water overnight in the goblet of your liquidizer. In the morning whizz them together until the almonds have turned into a fine pulp, and strain the milk through a fine sieve. The result is naturally sweet and excellent for drinking, while the pulp can be added to rice pudding.

Variation:
Try the same method with other nuts, such as brazils and cashews.

Home-made Ginger Tea with Lemon Zest

Pour a cupful of boiling water on to a teaspoon of grated fresh ginger and a teaspoon of fresh lemon zest shreds. Leave to infuse for 5 minutes, then strain and drink. This is an excellent drink if you feel a cold coming on, or if you have a tummy upset.

Dietary supplements

It is not essential to take dietary supplements with the Waterfall Diet. Many people believe that all of us get all the vitamins and minerals we need from a good, healthy diet, and this is true provided that you don't have extra needs due to absorption problems as discussed on p. 126. If you already eat a healthy diet but still have some of the signs of nutritional deficiencies listed below, perhaps you are one of those people with extra high needs.

Whether or not you fall into this category I generally advise taking a supplement programme, at least during Phase I of the Waterfall Diet, as an insurance policy. I often explain this in terms of a business which has become bankrupt – one that does not have enough cash to pay all the bills. As far as the human body is concerned, substitute nutrients for cash, and health problem for bankruptcy. Even in a bankrupt business there is still some cash around, but meanwhile machinery has been sold off to pay creditors, and stock levels have dwindled to nothing. You can get a bankrupt business going again, but you need a large inflow of capital. I view vitamin and mineral and other dietary supplements as that extra capital.

Symptoms of Various Nutritional Deficiencies

- Bad skin or hair
- Birth defects in the newborn
- Bouts of depression unrelated to external events
- Chronic tiredness
- Deteriorating memory
- Eye and ear problems
- Fluid retention (some types)
- Heart (artery) disease
- Hyperactivity in children
- Increasing chemical sensitivity or food intolerance
- Increasing mental confusion
- Infertility
- Kidney stones
- Menopausal symptoms
- Mental illness (in combination with extreme stress)
- Osteoporosis (brittle bone disease)
- Period pains
- Premenstrual syndrome
- Senile behaviour
- Spasms
- Tendency to catch colds and flu
- Tendency to suffer from thrush
- Uncharacteristic mood swings and unusual aggression

When using dietary supplements, it is usually a good idea to take a multivitamin and multimineral preparation as a foundation. This helps to prevent imbalances caused by taking one nutrient on its own for too long. Check the labels so that the combination of products you take provides approximately the following:

Recommended Basic Multivitamin and Mineral Formula

Vitamin A	7500 iu[1]
Vitamin B1, B2, B6	25–50 mg
Vitamin B12	50 mcg
Niacin (vitamin B3)	50 mg
Folic acid	400 mcg
Pantothenic acid (vitamin B5)	50 mg
Vitamin C	100 mg
Vitamin D	200 iu [2]
Vitamin E	50 iu [3]
Boron	2 mg
Chromium	50 mcg
Copper	0.5 mg (500 mcg)
Iron	5 mg
Manganese	5 mg
Selenium	50 mcg
Zinc	10 mg
Evening primrose, borage or blackcurrant seed oil [4]	250 mg
Fish oil [5]	250 mg

Values given for minerals are elemental (i.e. for the mineral only, not for compounds such as magnesium oxide or chromium picolinate, which may contain only a small proportion of the mineral itself). Check the labels on your supplement to ensure that the manufacturer also gives elemental values.

For children, reduce dosages in proportion to body weight.

The above dosages are considered safe in pregnancy.

Magnesium (approx 100–200 mg/a day) will normally need to be taken separately, since adding the required amount to a multinutrient formula would make each tablet or capsule too bulky. Many people also take additional vitamin C, up to 1000 or 2000 mg a day, to help combat pollution and prevent infections. If these amounts of vitamin C look very large to you, remember that most mammals produce (proportionally) much more vitamin C than this in their own bodies every day. Humans are missing the last stage in the liver enzyme process which produces vitamin C from glucose.

1. One iu = 0.3 micrograms (mcg or ug) of vitamin A
2. One iu = 0.025 micrograms of vitamin D
3. One iu = approx 1.5 milligrams (mg) of vitamin E
4. The active nutritional ingredient in these oils is gamma linolenic acid (GLA)
5. The active nutritional ingredients in these oils are eicosapentaenoic acid (EPA) and docosahexaenoic acid (DHA). Fish oil supplements are not the same as fish liver oils, which contain little EPA and DHA but are a good source of vitamin A.

The following herbs are rich in coumarins, flavonoids and other helpful nutrients:

- Ginkgo biloba
- Horse-chestnut
- Silymarin
- King's clover
- Gotu kola

Send a stamped addressed envelope for information to BCM Waterfall, London WC1N 3XX if you have any difficulties obtaining suitable vitamin, mineral or herbal formulas at reasonable cost, or visit www.waterfall.org.uk on the Internet.

Useful Addresses

International

The Lymphoedema Association of Australia
95 Cambridge Terrace, Malvern, SA 5061, Australia.
Tel +61 (8)8271 2198
Fax +61 (8)8271 8776
E-mail casley@enternet.com.au
Website: http://www.lymphoedema.org.au
A non-profit charity which supplies information to doctors on improving the effectiveness of lymphoedema treatments. Handles enquiries from all over the world. Publications for patients also available, including guides and videos for self-massage and exercising. The web site gives much useful information, including suppliers of coumarin in different countries, and therapists who have been trained by the LAA.

Hamilton Laboratories
GPO Box 7, Adelaide, SA 5001, Australia
Fax +61 (8)232 1480.
Suppliers of Lodema®. If you cannot obtain it in your own country, this firm will supply it to any individual in any country for private use. Most countries will permit the importation of a medicine which is freely available in another country for the personal use of a single patient. But not all customs officers are aware of this! You do not need this product unless you have been diagnosed with lymphoedema by a doctor.

The Waterfall Diet Website

www.waterfall.org.uk

For more information, tips and help with other health problems.

United Kingdom

The Breakspear Hospital

Lord Alexander House, Waterhouse St, Hemel Hempstead, Herts. HP1 1DL

Tel: 01442 261333

International environmental medicine treatment unit, for laboratory diagnosis of chemical poisoning and environmental illness, and medically supervised nutritional detox programmes.

British Society for Allergy, Environmental and Nutritional Medicine

PO Box 28, Totton, Southampton, Hants, SO40 2ZA

A society of doctors who apply the principles of nutritional medicine and treat patients accordingly.

British Society for Mercury-Free Dentistry

1 Welbeck House, Welbeck St, London W1M 7HB

Send sae or international postal coupon for information.

Eating Disorders Association

Sackville Place, 44 Magdalen St, Norwich, Norfolk, NR3 1JE

Tel: 01603 621414

Provides help and guidance for those with eating disorders.

The Fresh Food Company

326 Portobello Rd, London W10 5RU Tel: 020 8969 0351

E-mail: organic@freshfood.co.uk

Internet: www.freshfood.co.uk

Nationwide deliveries of organic food and fresh fish, with large and interesting catalogue.

Health Interlink Ltd

Interlink House, 1a Crown St, Redbourn, Herts, AL3 7JX
Tel: 01582 794094
Can put you in touch with practitioners who make use of some of
the laboratory tests mentioned in this book.

Herbs of Grace

5a Lanwades Business Park, Kennett, Newmarket, Suffolk, CB8
7PN
Tel: 01638 750140
Mail order suppliers of dried clover blossoms.

The Nutri Centre

7 Park Crescent, London W1N 3HE
Tel: 020 7436 5122
Mail order suppliers of many dietary supplements, including,
magnesium taurate, n-acetyl cysteine (NAC), coenzyme Q10 and
other products mentioned in this book.

Society for the Promotion of Nutritional Therapy

BCM Box SPNT, London WC1N 3XX
Tel: 01825 872 921
E-mail: spnt@compuserve.com
Internet: http://visitweb.com/spnt
Send sae plus £1 to receive a list of your nearest registered nutritional
therapists in Great Britain. Nutritional therapists can help with a host
of ailments from migraine to skin problems, PMS, irritable bowel
syndrome and chronic tiredness. The SPNT is an educational and
campaigning organization with branches throughout the UK and
members in many foreign countries. Publishes quarterly journal
Nutritional Therapy Today for members. Factsheets and other publications also available, including *Clinical Pearls News*, which provides
monthly research summaries, and *Nutritional Influences on Illness*, an
excellent sourcebook of clinical research.
Send £16 (UK) £20 (Europe) or £24 (rest of the world) to join the
society for one year.

The Soil Association
Bristol House, 40–56 Victoria St, Bristol, BS1 6BY
Tel: 0117 929 3202
Contact for details of organic suppliers in your area.

The Vegan Society
Donald Watson House, 7 Battle Rd, St Leonards on Sea, East
Sussex, TN37 7AA
Tel: 01424 427393
Can provide scientific information written by qualified state-regis-
tered dieticians on the health and safety of diets free of dairy and
other animal produce.

United States
American Academy of Environmental Medicine
4510 W. 89th Street, Prairie Village, Kansas 66207
Tel: (913) 341 3625
Register of practitioners of environmental medicine.

American Association of Naturopathic Physicians
601 Valley St, Suite 105, Seattle, WA 98109
Tel: (206) 298 0125

American College of Advancement in Medicine
PO Box 3427, Laguna Hills, CA 92654
Tel: (714) 583 7666

American Environmental Health Foundation
8345 Walnut Hill Lane, Suite 200, Dallas, Texas 75231-4262
Tel: (214) 368 4132
Organization for the recognition and appropriate treatment of
environmental illness. Books and publications available.

American Preventive Medical Association
275 Millway, PO Box 732, Barnstable, ME 02630
Tel: (508) 362 4343
Register of practitioners sympathetic to a natural approach to medicine.

Great Smokies Laboratory
63 Zillicoa St, Asheville, NC 28801-1074
Tel: (704) 253 0621
Internet: www.gsdl.com
Can put you in touch with practitioners who use some of the tests mentioned in this book.

HealthComm International
PO Box 1729, Gig Harbor, Washington 98335
Tel: (206) 851 3943
Provides educational materials for healthcare practitioners interested in functional and nutritional medicine.

IT Services
3301 Alta Arden #2, Sacramento, California 95825
Tel: (916) 483 1085
Publishers of *Clinical Pearls News*, an excellent monthly summary of the latest natural medicine research.

Linus Pauling Institute
440 Page Mill Rd, Palo Alto, CA 94306-2031
Centre for research into vitamin C.

Australia
Australian College of Nutritional and Environmental Medicine
13 Hilton St, Beaumaris, Victoria 3193
Tel: +61 (3)9589 6088
For a referral service for all conventionally trained GPs and specialists who are interested in a wider and more natural approach to illness.

Australian Natural Therapists Association
Taren Point, PO Box 2517, Sydney 2232

Canada
International Society for Orthomolecular Medicine
16 Florence Avenue, Toronto, M2N 1E9
Tel: (416) 733 2117
An international society for health professionals.

New Zealand
Association of Natural Therapies
81 Forrest Hill Road, Milford, Auckland

Society of Naturopaths
Box 19183, Auckland 7

How Did You Get On With The Waterfall Diet?

Much of the information in this book has never before been presented to people trying to lose weight. If we are to bring about any changes in the way weight problems are treated in the health-care system, research is essential. The best way to stimulate interest for the funding of such research is to show doctors and dieticians a wealth of case histories.

If you have read this book and tried the Waterfall Diet, your feedback would be very much appreciated. To help others, could I ask you to complete the following questionnaire? If you do not want to cut it out of the book, please feel free to write your answers on a separate piece of paper.

Waterfall Diet Questionnaire

1. How much did you weigh before starting the Waterfall Diet
   _____?

2. How much do you weigh now?_____

3. Were you on a calorie-controlled diet before beginning the Waterfall Diet? YES/NO If so, how many calories per day?
   _____

4. How long did you spend on Phase I of the Waterfall Diet?
   _____

5. Did you complete Phase II of the Waterfall Diet? YES/NO

6. How easy did you find the Waterfall Diet? (please tick as appropriate)
   - ❑ Impossible, I gave up after _____ days because

   _____

   _____

   _____

   - ❑ Very difficult, but I was able to persevere
   - ❑ Difficult, but becoming easier as I got used to it
   - ❑ No more difficult than other diets I have tried
   - ❑ Relatively easy compared with other diets I have tried
   - ❑ Very easy

7. How successful have you found the Waterfall Diet compared with a normal calorie-controlled diet?
   - ❑ Much more successful
   - ❑ About the same
   - ❑ Less successful
   - ❑ Not effective at all

8. What type of fluid retention do the questionnaires suggest you had (tick as appropriate)?
   - ❑ Allergic
   - ❑ Protein deficiency
   - ❑ Kidney stress
   - ❑ Prescription medicines
   - ❑ Internal pollution
   - ❑ Capillary or lymphatic problems
   - ❑ Vitamin or mineral deficiencies

9. Do you think doctors and dieticians should be trained in the principles of the Waterfall Diet? YES/NO

10. Do you have any other comments about the Waterfall Diet?

_____

_____

_____

_____

_____

_____

_____

Your name and address (optional)

_____

_____

_____

_____

Thank you so much for your assistance. Please send your answers to:

Linda Lazarides
BCM Waterfall
London WC1N 3XX

Website = www.waterfall.org.uk

Linda Lazarides regrets that queries about the diet or about weight loss cannot be answered individually, but all questions and comments that may be of help and interest to others will be covered in forthcoming editions of *The Waterfall Diet*.

Index